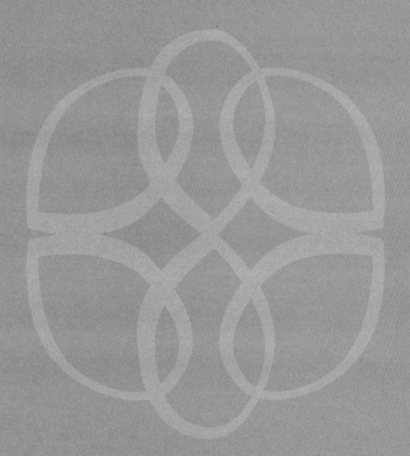

Health and Beauty from the Rainforest

Malaysian Traditions of Ramuan

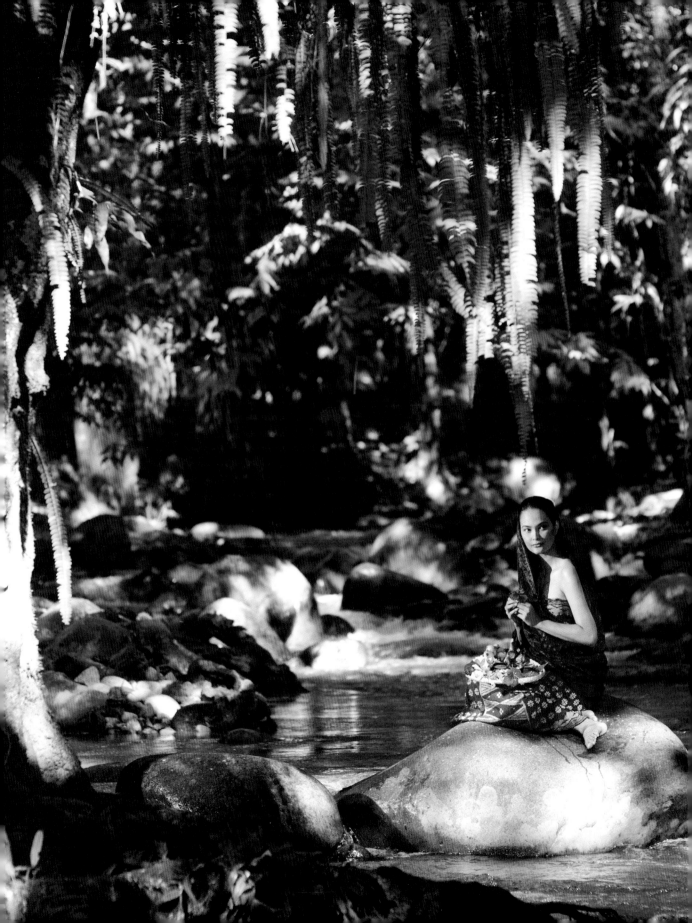

Health and Beauty from the Rainforest

Malaysian Traditions of Ramuan

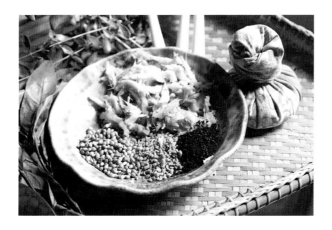

Editor-in-chief
Gerard Bodeker

Editors
Hood Salleh
Ruzy Suliza Hashim
Christof Jaenicke
Joerg Gruenwald
Zurinawati Zainal Abidin

Photographer
S.C. Shekar

Editions D*idier* M*illet*

Editorial Team

Editor-in-chief
Gerard Bodeker

Editors
Hood Salleh
Ruzy Suliza Hashim
Christof Jaenicke
Joerg Gruenwald
Zurinawati Zainal Abidin

Project Directors
Matthias Miller
Tengku Shahrir Tengku Adnan

Project Coordinator
Noorsyarida Mohd Sapiai

Contributors
Daniel Baskaran
Dorai Raja
Andrew Forbes
Haliza Mohd Riji
Hamzah Abu Al-Haj
Lee Jok Keng
Musa Yaacob
Sairani Mohd Sa'ad
Sharifah Anisah Syed Agil Barakbah
Zainatul Shuhaida Abdul Rahman

Photographer

S.C. Shekar

Acknowledgements

We wish to thank all of the contributors as well as the
Ayurvedium Medispa, Badan Warisan Malaysia, Forest Research
Institute Malaysia (FRIM), Kim Inglis, YTL Corporation Berhad, Federal
Land Development Authority (FELDA), Nona Roguy Spa, Pathmavathy
Suresh, and Tourism Selangor Sdn Bhd.

Medical Disclaimer

The information published or contained in this book is based on traditional cultural
knowledge and practice and is not intended to replace the services of a physician.
Health-related content is provided for informational purposes only and shall not be
construed in any manner whatsoever to be a substitute or an option or alternative
for professional medical advice. Readers are advised and recommended to consult
a physician in all matters relating to their health, and particularly in respect to any
symptoms that may require diagnosis or medical attention.

Publishing Team

Publisher	Didier Millet
General Manager	Charles Orwin
Editorial Director	Timothy Auger
Project Manager	Martin Cross
Project Coordinator	Wong Ee Laine
Assistant Project Coordinator	Joane Sharmila
Stylist	Li Yuemin
Copy Editor	William Citrin
Studio Manager	Yusri bin Din
Designer	Vani Nadaraju
Production Manager	Sin Kam Cheong

Text and photographs © Biotropics Malaysia Berhad
Book design © Editions Didier Millet, 2009

Editions Didier Millet
25, Jalan Pudu Lama, 50200 Kuala Lumpur, Malaysia
Tel: 03-2031 3805 Fax: 03-2031 6298
E-mail: edmbooks@edmbooks.com.my

Website: www.edmbooks.com

First published 2009
Reprinted 2009

Editions Didier Millet Pte Ltd
121, Telok Ayer Street, #03-01, Singapore 068590
Tel: 65-6324 9260 Fax: 65-6324 9261
E-mail:edm@edmbooks.com.sg

Color separation by SC Graphic
Printed by Tien Wah Press

ISBN 978-981-4217-91-0

Page 2: Ramuan for health and beauty are derived from Malaysia's diverse
rainforest environment.
Page 3: A selection of *ramuan* ingredients in a tray.
Opposite: Limes, roses and chrysanthemums are common ingredients used in Indian
floral baths.
Page 6: Herbal tea is regularly consumed by Chinese to promote health.
Page 7 (from top): Materials used in the Malay tradition of *melenggang perut* or 'swaying
of the abdomen'; Indian floral bath; *nasi ulam*; Chinese herbs; Malay floral bath.
Pages 8 and 9: Common ingredients used in *ramuan* for health and beauty.

(A wholly owned subsidiary of Khazanah Nasional Berhad)

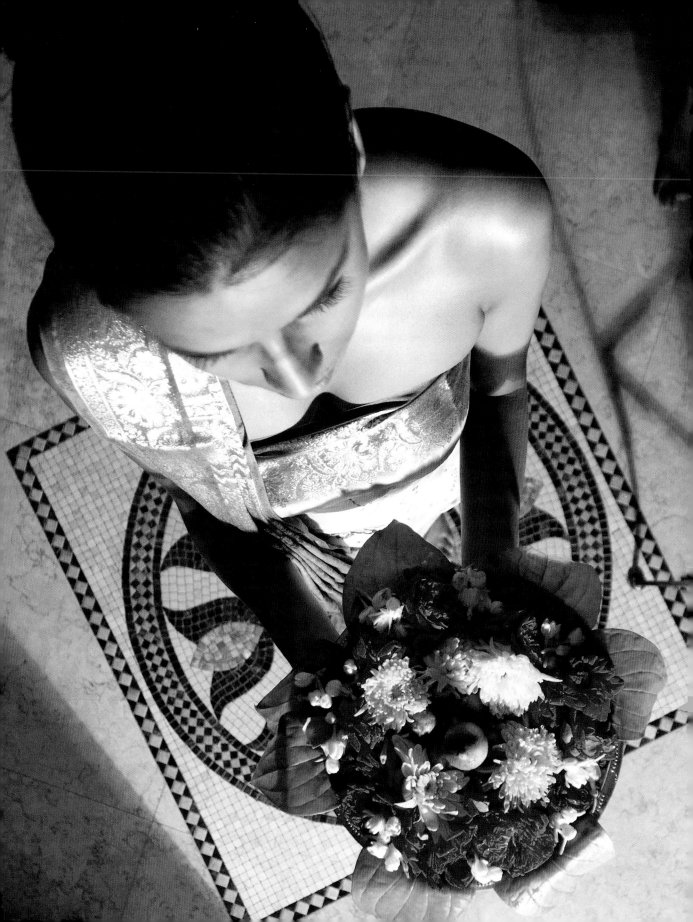

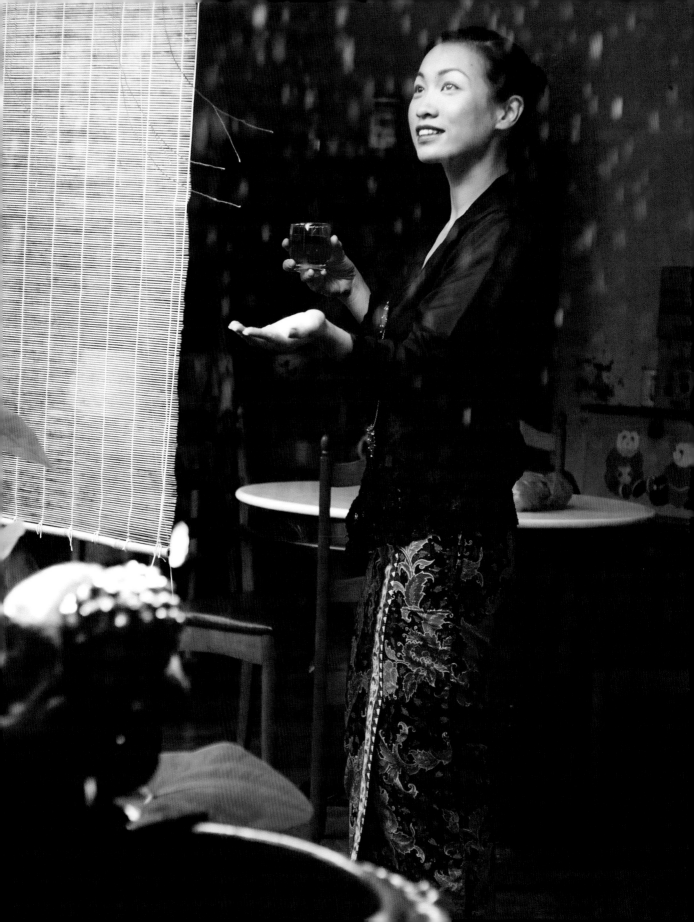

Contents

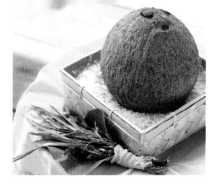

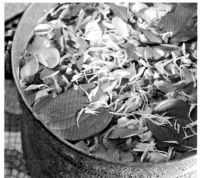

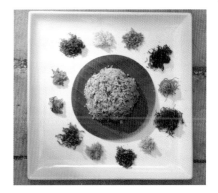

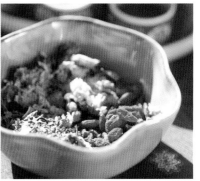

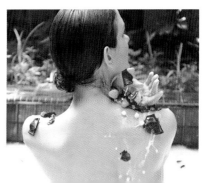

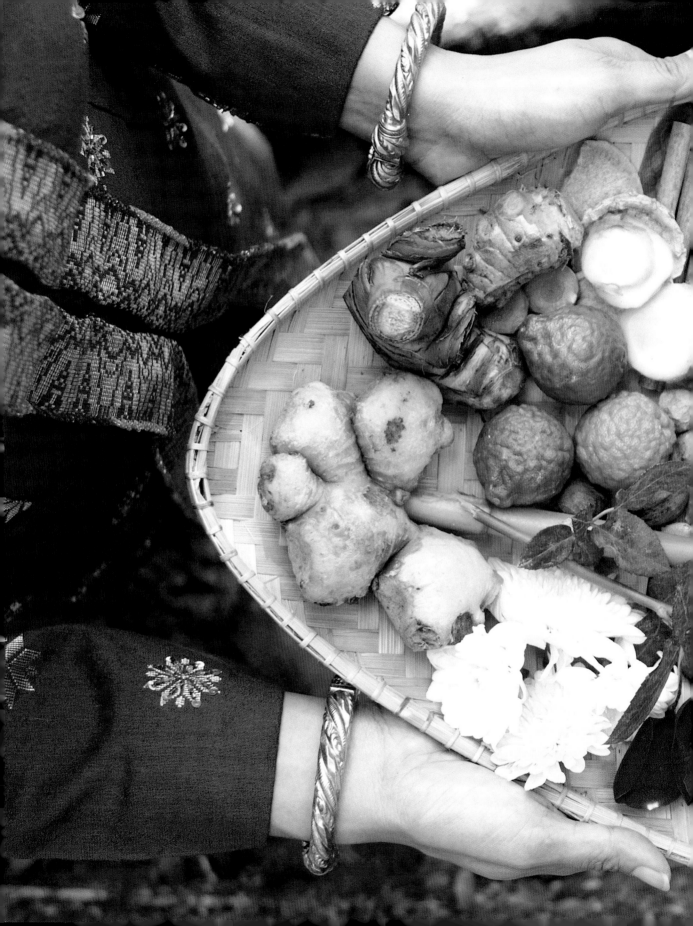

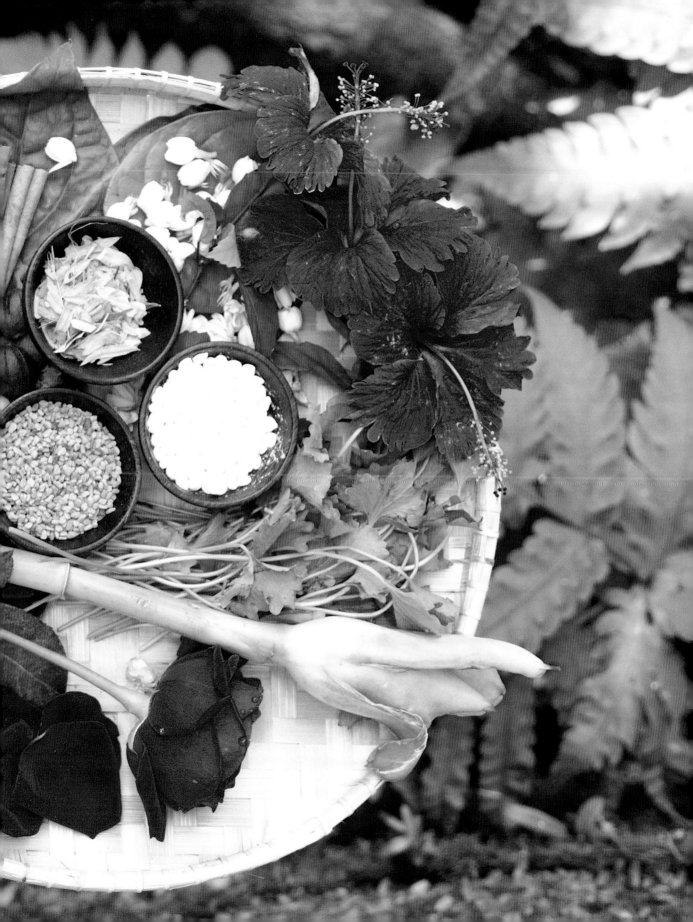

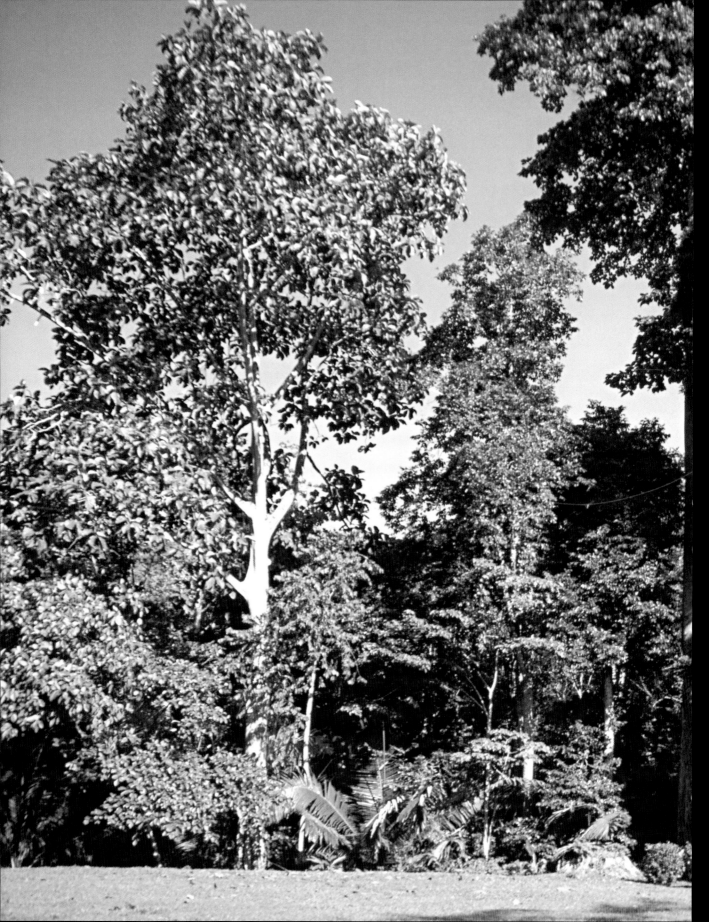

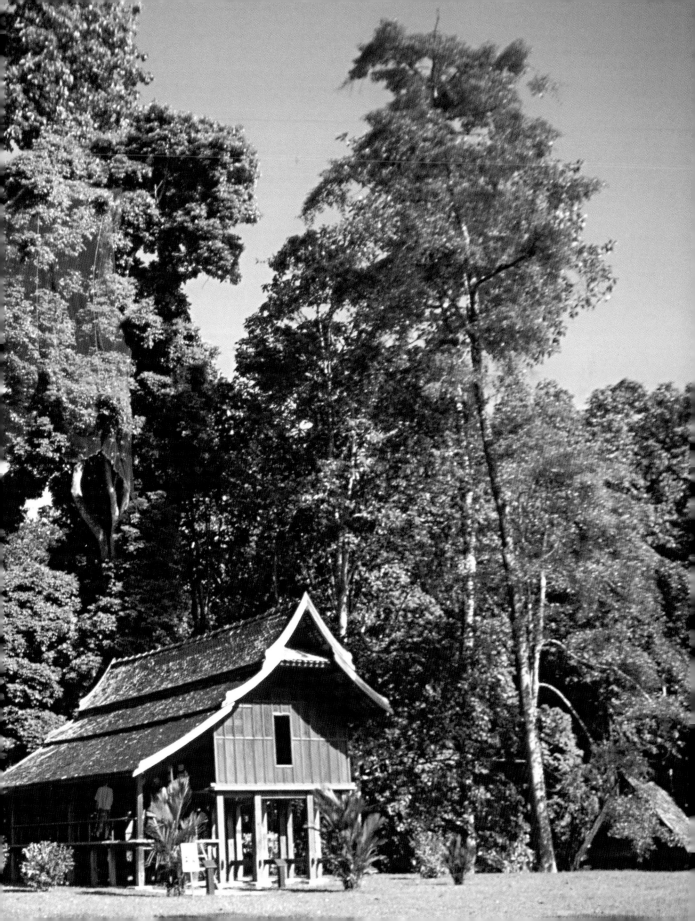

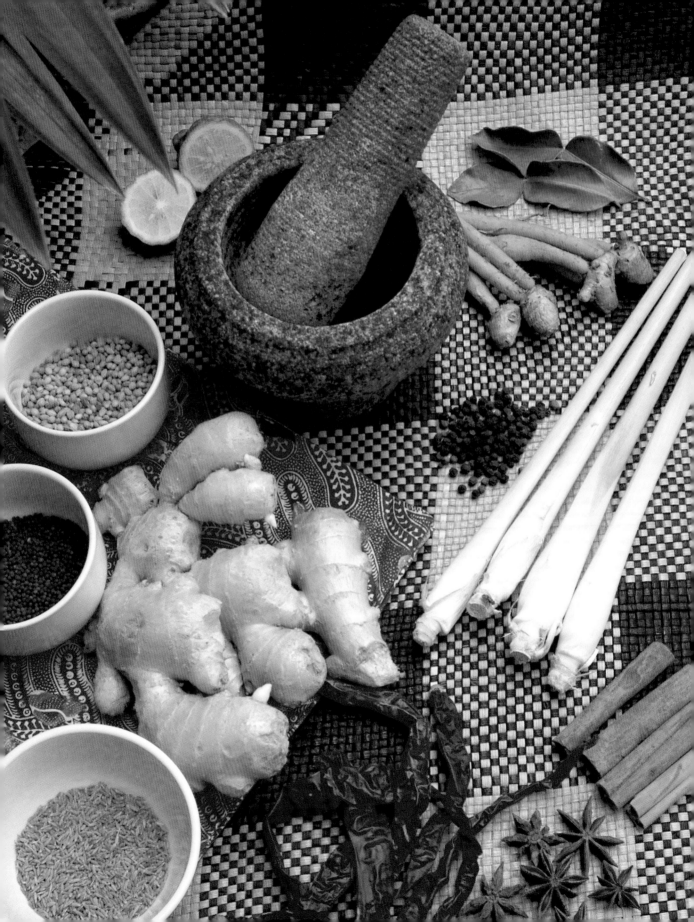

Introduction

*Nature lies at the heart of Asian wellness traditions.
Extract the healing essences of indigenous herbs, leaves,
flowers and roots and the blessings are manifold:
a burst of energy, a clear complexion, a feeling of inner
tranquility. The ancients in Malaysia knew this—and
much more—all along. It's time now to share their
age-old wisdom with the world.*

A healing mixture of medicinal plants and plant parts is referred to in the Malay language as *ramuan*. The word *ramuan* also denotes ingredients used for cooking. With multiple potent properties, including use in food, *ramuan* is seen as a force for healing, beauty and vitality.

In this ancient tropical land, strategically located to the north of the Indonesian Archipelago and Singapore, and reaching as far as Thailand, medicine and food are intertwined and interchangeable. Both are part and parcel of the daily process of seeking and maintaining balance—a concept considered vital for overall wellness.

Previous pages Malaysia's rainforests have played a vital role in shaping and influencing local traditions and customs.

Opposite *Ramuan*, comprising a mixture of ingredients, is a force for healing and beauty.

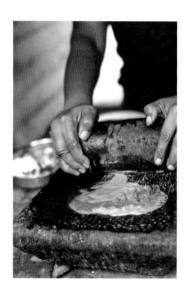

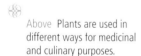

Above Plants are used in different ways for medicinal and culinary purposes.

Below For centuries, the Orang Asli have followed a lifestyle that relies on the bounty of local rainforests.

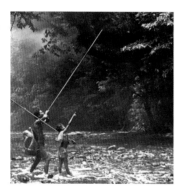

Fortunately, the source of *ramuan*—Malaysia's rainforests—is close at hand. Plants can be picked, mashed, cooked, consumed and applied at all times of the year. Originating over 130 million years ago in the Pleistocene Era, these rainforests are among the oldest on earth. Due to the extent of the biological diversity of its rainforests, Malaysia has been recognized as one of 12 global mega diversity areas. While the rest of the world went through eras of cooling and warming over millions of years, Malaysia's geographical position on the equator has meant that temperatures have remained more or less constant over millennia.

Surrounded by oceans that have provided enough moisture to deposit heavy monsoonal rains—around 200 centimeters (79 inches) each year—and temperatures varying from 20° to 35° Celsius (70° to 100° Fahrenheit), the region has consistently supported forests over tens of millions of years.

Rainforest Peoples and Cultures

In such a land, it is not surprising to find numerous myths and legends about nature and the origins of life. The country's indigenous inhabitants see the forests as living entities. Rich with character and power, the rainforests are respected, feared, appeased and lived from. Both a source of danger and a source of healing, they provide food and shelter—and also mystical protection. Similarly, the oceans and islands surrounding them are imbued with fabled princesses, dragons, beauty, heroism and quests that, to this day, endure as part of the fabric of modern legend and national identity.

Ramuan—the deliberate and intelligent bringing together of ingredients—is a mixture that brings balance and health. Analogously, the term can be used to characterize the mix of the more than 60 ethnic indigenous groups of Malaysia, and the wider group of Malays, Chinese and Indians who make up today's Malaysian society. Common to all of the people of modern Malaysia are deep cultural ties to the healing traditions of their ancestors. These traditions draw on and involve a

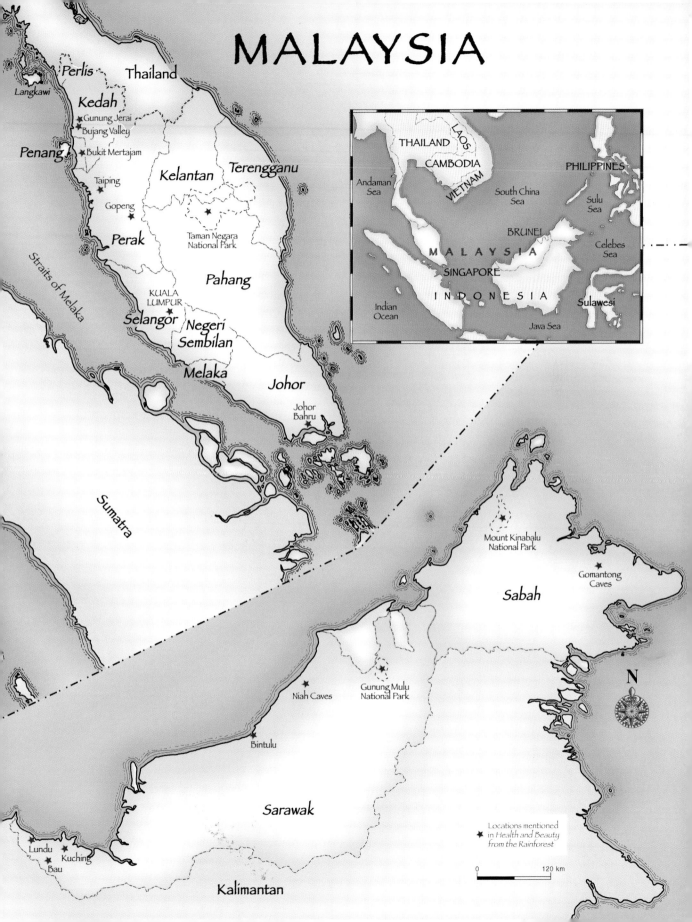

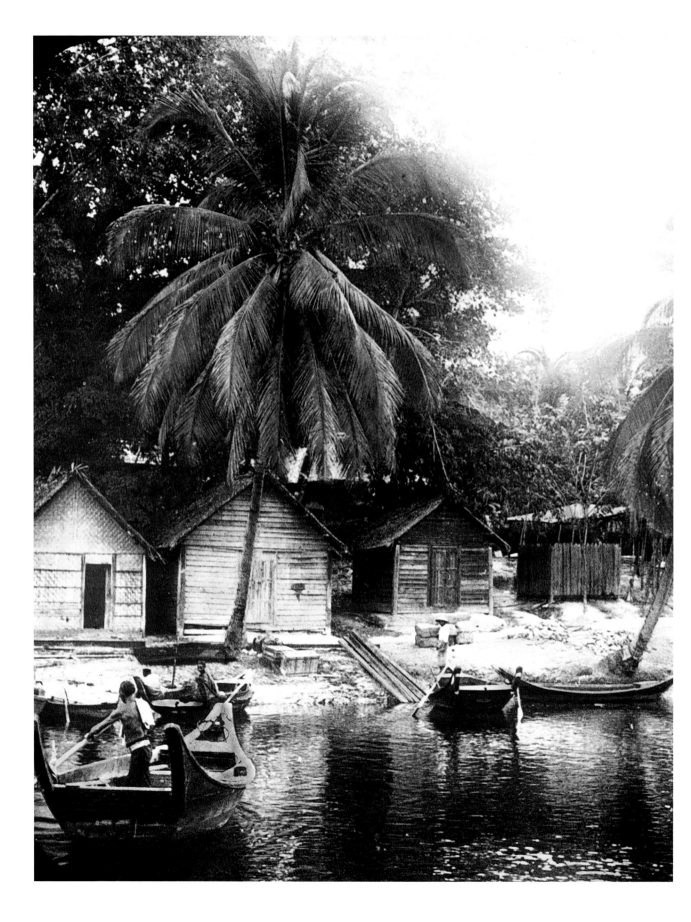

deep respect for the plants from the ancient rainforests. These plants are conserved and cultivated as well as utilized. They are prepared according to ancestral wisdom and Asian theories of natural science about the deeper principles of nature, such as temperature (hot and cold), taste (sweet, sour, salty and bitter), and touch (dry, damp, rough and soft).

Globalization in the Ancient World

The Malays—the majority community of Malaysia representing around 60 percent of the population—were originally seafaring people who settled on the Malay Peninsula as early as 1000 BCE. Recognized as a branch of the Austronesian peoples, their lineage may be traced back to what is present-day Taiwan at least 5,000 years. Between 5,000 and 2,500 years BCE, a large-scale migration out of southern China began and, by way of dugout canoes, fanned out across Southeast Asia, settling extraordinarily widely—from the Philippines and Polynesia, through Borneo and Sumatra, to the Malay Peninsula, and beyond.

Already at home with transnational exchange through their migration and trading patterns within Asia, the Malays became part of a global network approximately 2,000 years ago with the emergence of at least one major trading port on the west coast of the Malay Peninsula.

A natural point of anchor for trading vessels sailing from India on the monsoon winds, this port offered ships a break in their journey en route to Indonesia, Vietnam and, ultimately, China. The crew and their passengers would rest in a flourishing port in what is now the Malaysian state of Kedah (see page 136). In early times, this bountiful port, with its large harbor, was known variously as 'Suvarnabhumi' (or 'golden land' in Sanskrit), 'Kadaram' in Tamil, 'Jiecha' in Chinese and 'Kalah' to early Arab navigators. Ships from as far west as the Mediterranean knew of the port, and as early as 150 CE, the Greek geographer Ptolemy, echoing the Sanskrit name, styled the Malay Peninsula 'Aurea Chersonesus' or 'the golden peninsula'.

Opposite Malay village in a coconut grove, 1920s.

Below A 13th-century map of Southeast Asia taken from Ptolemy's *Geographike Huphegesis* or 'Guide to Geography'. The Malay Peninsula is labeled 'Aurea Chersonesus' which translates as 'the golden peninsula'.

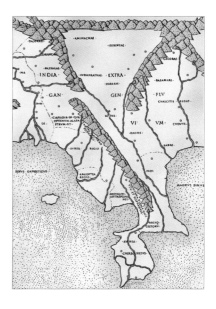

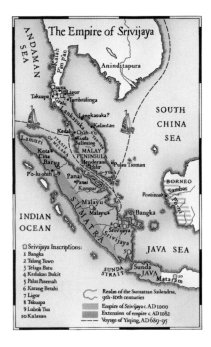

The Empire of Srivijaya

Srivijaya Inscriptions:
1 Bangka
2 Talang Tewo
3 Telaga Batu
4 Kedukan Bukit
5 Palas Pasemah
6 Karang Berahi
7 Ligor
8 Takuapa
9 Lubok Tua
10 Kalasan

Realm of the Sumatran Sailendras, 9th–10th centuries
Empire of Srivijaya c. AD 1000
Extension of empire c. AD 1082
Voyage of Yiqing, AD 689–95

Above Map depicting the extent of the Srivijayan Empire in the Malay Peninsula and Sumatra.

Below This bronze Buddha statue, dating from the 6th to 7th century CE, was found in Kedah.

Opposite Perak women in traditional Malay dress and jewelry in the early 1900s. The lady seated was the wife of the state's ruler Abdul Jalil (r. 1916–18).

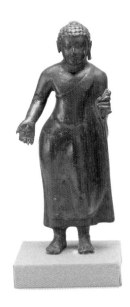

Chinese scholars en route to India to study Buddhist scriptures stopped there for weeks and sometimes months at a time. Their diary records from the 3rd and 6th centuries reinforce Indian and Greek reports of the land as a place of abundance and ease, refinement, culture and beauty, a vast port settlement where civilized living was the norm and international trade the lifeblood. A veritable bridge between the East and the West, Kadaram flourished for more than 1,000 years under royal houses that had marriage ties to Vietnam, Cambodia and Indonesia as well as India and China.

Globalization—a contemporary term for an ancient phenomenon—was very much part of the way of life in this ancient Malay world. With traders from the East and West came others who brought knowledge. Scholars, physicians and monks traveled the long sea journey in each direction—from India to China via Kadaram and other historic ports in the Srivijayan and Cambodian Empires and from China to India and the Persian Gulf via the same entrepôts and tributaries.

The early Hindu-Buddhist kingdoms of the Malay Peninsula would have drawn on both Ayurvedic and Siddha knowledge that came with cultural and spiritual influences from India (see pages 131–149). Similarly, ingredients commonly used in India would be replaced with Malay *ramuan* found here.

In ancient times, the medicinal properties of plants and trees from the Malaysian rainforests were among the precious gifts offered in tribute by the Raja of Kadaram to the Chinese Emperor. When Muslim traders arrived on the Malay Peninsula in the 10th century, bringing with them Islam and Arabic medicine, there was a shift in tradition and governance from the courts of Indianized rajas to a more Arabic system of rule—the sultanates.

Today, modern-day Malaysian language and culture reflect these rich historical antecedents. Enduring traditions, such as wedding ceremonies and other customs in the royal courts of Malaysia's current sultans, hark back to ancient Indian practices. Religion, some aspects of the language, and methods of trade and monetary exchange show the enduring presence of early

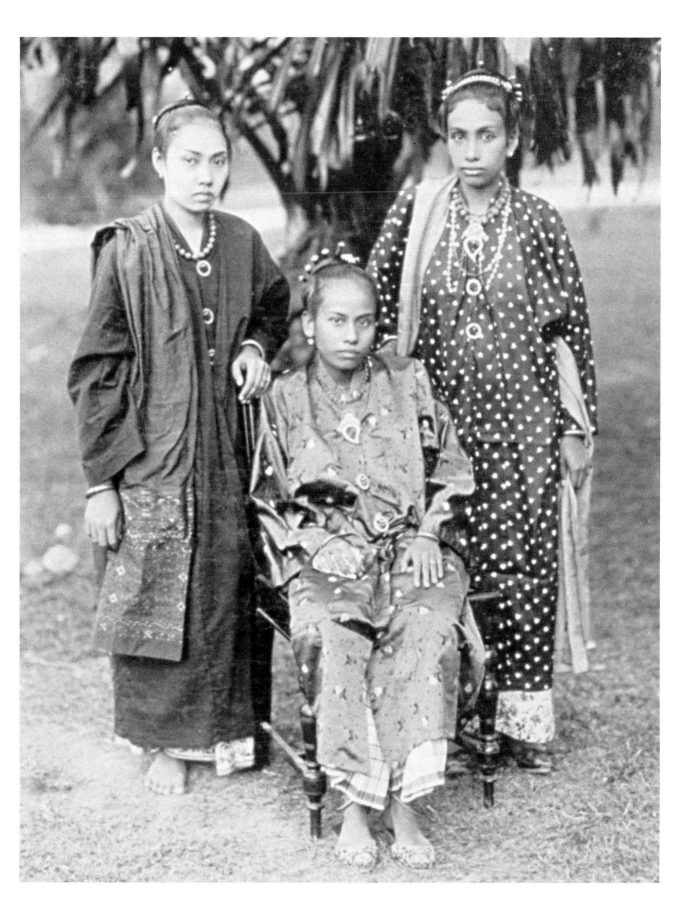

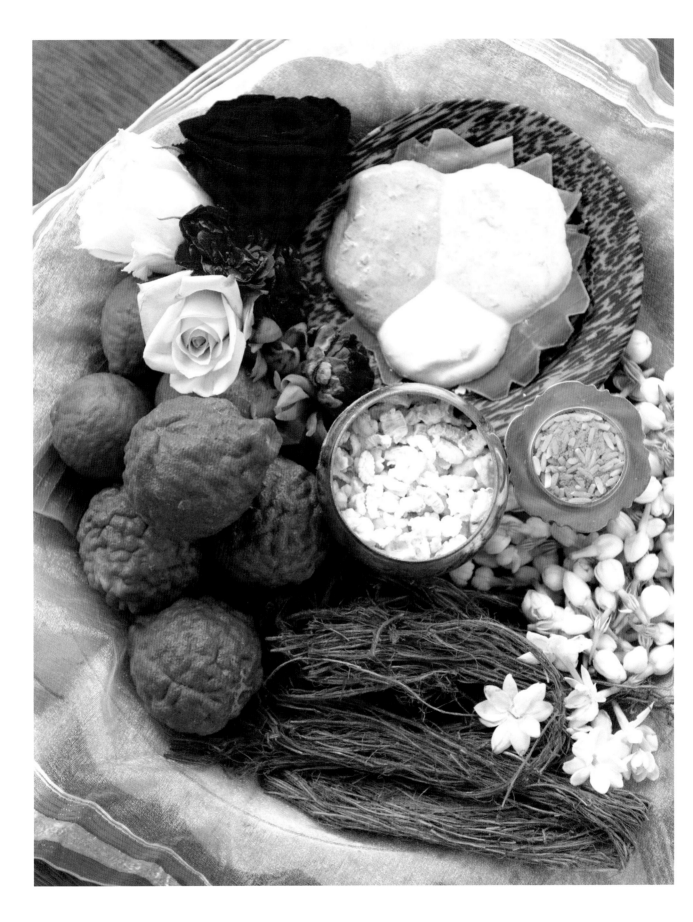

Arabic influences. And Malaysian society, with its mix of peoples—Orang Asli, Malays, Indians, Chinese and immigrants from all over Asia and beyond—remains consistent with its ancient roots. What a *ramuan* of culture, genetic influences and lifestyles! Small wonder that Malaysia's overseas tourist campaigns position the country as 'truly Asia'.

Traditions of Health and Beauty

Taking a lifestyle approach to wellness, Malaysian traditions look beyond health to focus on improving one's quality of life and the different needs of men and women. In the Malay world, inner and outer health and beauty go hand in hand.

Long before today's surge of 'cosmeceuticals', where beauty products are imbued with nutritional and pharmacological properties, *ramuan* preparations made from rainforest ingredients for women herbal masks and scrubs, flower baths, scented steams and herbal oils—were used to create beauty from health-giving effects. For men, aware that energy is key to overall health, *ramuan* treatments focused on male vitality and vigor.

Today, scientific studies are beginning to validate the efficacy of some of these traditional formulations and the country is becoming more aware of the therapeutic and commercial potential of the *ramuan* tradition. For example, a Malay-themed massage program has been introduced in a national hospital and a local university offers a diploma course in Malay massage, known as *urut*.

Reflecting this surge of interest in Malaysia's pan-Asian cultural heritage, Malaysian spas of a high international caliber are offering Malay healing treatments, Malaysian Chinese and Peranakan secret practices of health and beauty, and Ayurvedic approaches to health, wellbeing and balance. Drawing on these multicultural historical practices, many of which originated thousands of years ago and possibly thousands of miles distant from Malaysia, and combining them with indigenous healing wisdom adds more richness to the mix.

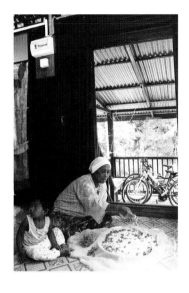

Opposite One of many *ramuan* compositions used in the Malay tradition.

Above *Bedak sejuk* (a cooling herbal talc) prepared the traditional way in a *kampung* in Bukit Mertajam, Penang.

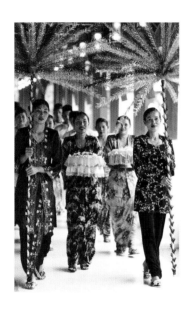

Above Floral bath procession at a five-star spa in Terengganu.

Opposite Malay practices and traditions are finding their way into modern Malaysian spas.

For example, at a five-star spa in the northern state of Terengganu, a ceremony is conducted where spa ingredients or *ramuan* are carried in a musical procession by village people, beating drums, invoking blessings on the ingredients, and drawing water from vessels that in turn are filled with waters from rivers and sources of healing. Once these are collected and combined, a personal attendant slowly pours this floral water over the bathing guest. Then, while the guest stands deep in an outdoor immersion pool, the attendant, invoking wishes of abundance and fullness, again pours this special water in libation over the head and shoulders of the guest.

The wellness environment, then, begins in advance of the actual therapies that ensue. Mind, emotions and receptivity are heightened in the process; the guest feels royal, special and deeply cared for. The treatment draws on the best of nature's healing secrets, applied sincerely with heart-warming sentiments from local tradition, for an experience of inner enjoyment and growth. The Malay philosophy invoked here is known as *suci murni* and it emphasizes purity of spirit, health and wellbeing.

With both village and royal Malay practices finding their way into the world of spas, many Malaysian spas are now being recognized by the wellness world internationally. Add to this Ayurvedic, Siddha, Unani and traditional Chinese medicinal therapies, and it is easy to see how much Malaysia has to offer.

Innovation in the spa industry, therapies backed up by scientific trials, formulations presented in a manner more familiar to foreigners, and an ancient culture of wellness are compelling reasons to visit the country. Visitors to Malaysia are coming for exactly that—Asian tropical rainforests, Asian cultures and food, Asian hospitality and lifestyle, and, increasingly, Asian wellness.

This book delves into the history of these rich traditions. It examines the rituals, the botanicals, the people and the cultures, and with the benefit of a contemporary perspective, cuts through myth to fact and actuality. Malaysia's *ramuan*, with its healing and beautifying powers, is finally receiving global attention. It is richly deserved and deeply fascinating.

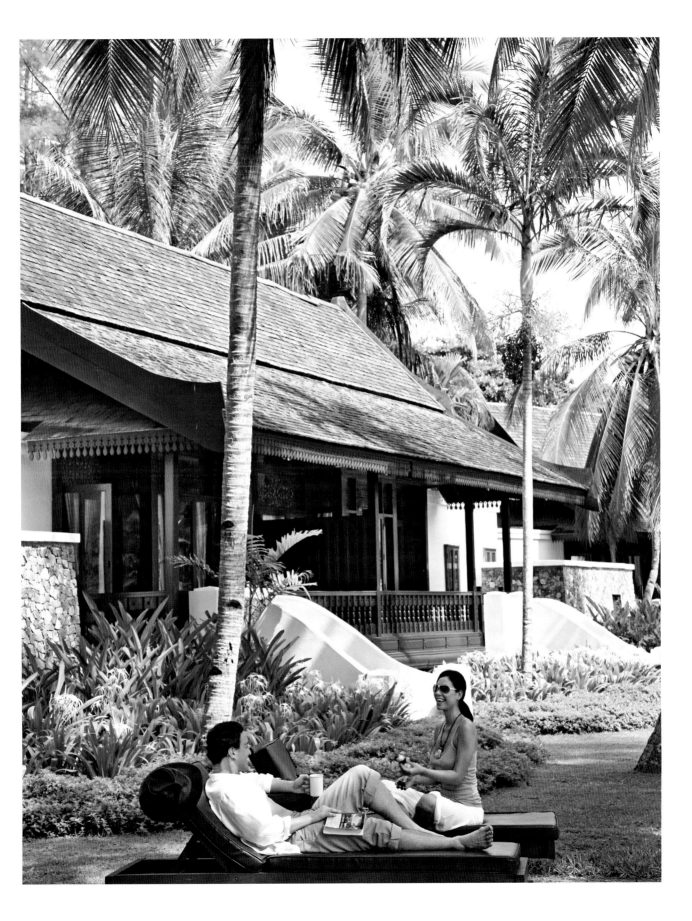

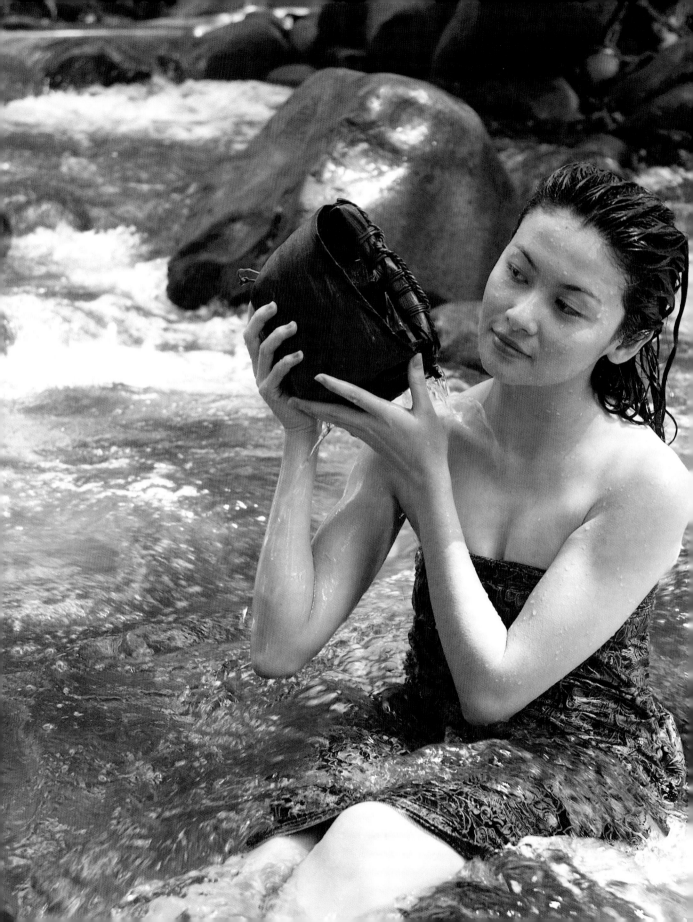

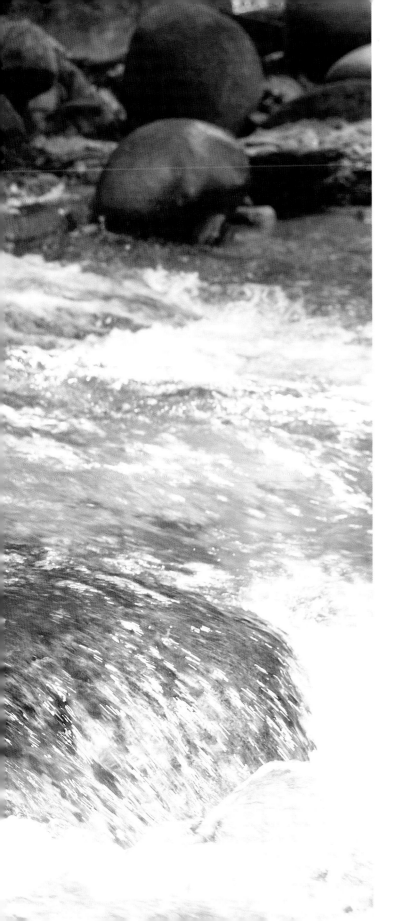

Health and Beauty in Malay Society

Advocating balance, moderation and a holistic approach, traditional Malay healing focuses on attuning the body's energies with the rhythms of nature. A mix of different traditions and cultures, Malay healing emphasizes the idea of inter-connectedness with the environment—what resides within us also goes on around us. It also lays stress on the maintenance of a vigorous mind–body–soul balance and the strong link between internal health and outer appearance. Primarily revolving around healthcare in the family, there are specific formulae and rituals for every stage in a person's life. All rely on the bounty and beauty of nature.

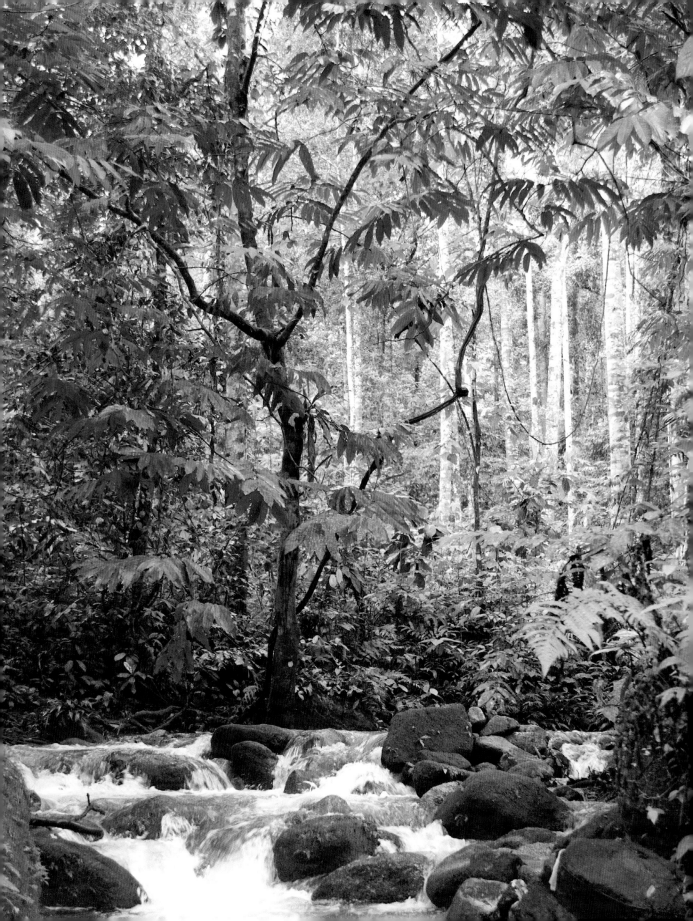

A Life in Balance
The Principles of Ramuan

The concepts and beliefs underlying the Malaysian system of *ramuan* are based on more than 2,000 years of investigation, knowledge and practice. Its roots are found in both oral and written traditions, combining the teachings and wisdom of early Orang Asli populations with that of the Malay traders and voyagers who first began to settle and develop the region several millennia ago. In recent millennia, to this already rich blend was added knowledge adopted and adapted from three separate belief systems—those of India, China and the Arab world, the last of which had been influenced by early Greek and Roman precepts. In other words, *ramuan* is an ancient and sophisticated system founded in the Malay world's traditions, but strongly influenced by the various cultures and peoples who have traded, fought, settled, inter-married and otherwise traversed or settled in the region over the centuries.

A useful analogy might be a lacquered vase: the first layer contains the Orang Asli and Malay traditions, which are over-layered in turn by veneers of varying thickness from the Indo-Buddhist civilizations of South Asia, the Islamic civilization of Arabia and the Sinitic civilization of China and East Asia. And, as if this were not enough, from the 16th century, European influences were also transmitted to the region by nations as diverse as Portugal, Spain, Holland, France and Great Britain.

Previous pages *Mandi sungai*, or bathing in a river.

Opposite Gunung Bunga Buah in Pahang. Malaysia's rainforests provide precious medicinal plants and natural resources.

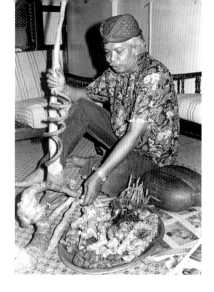

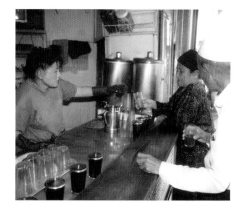

Above A *dukun* displays some herbs and plant roots used in the making of traditional Malay medicines.

Below Malay customers buying herbal drinks from a Chinese vendor in Johor Bahru. Malaysians benefit from one another's traditions.

Opposite *Ramuan* is an integration of ingredients.

Key Personnel: 'Doctors' and 'Patients'

Practitioners of Malay traditional medicine can be divided into several categories: the *bomoh* or medicine man; the *dukun* or soothsayer and herbalist; the *pawang* or shaman; and the *bidan* or midwife. These people generally gained their expertise by studying and learning for many years from skilled practitioners.

While bomoh, dukun and pawang are called on in particular cases of illness, bidan serve their community in the fields of general health and sexual matters. Although they specialize in ante-natal, delivery and post-natal care, they may be consulted in the case of common illnesses and for beauty advice. Their remedies include both internal consumption and external application of mixtures of medicinal herbs and plants (or *ramuan*).

As the Malaysian population today comprises a diverse mix of ethnic groups, it is not only the Malays who benefit from Malay herbal traditions. Chinese patients may consult a Malay bomoh in the same way that Malays go to a Chinese *sinseh* shop to restore their *yin-yang* or inner energy and physical balance. Similarly, foot reflexology centers are patronized by all ethnic groups. Malays also make use of Ayurvedic and Unani medicine typically found in urban areas. This is one of the underlying strengths of *ramuan*: the willingness of any one Malaysian ethnic group to believe, to a greater or lesser extent, in the potency and efficacy of the health and wellness practices of another. To give two examples: Malay healers have long recognized the usefulness of ginseng—adopted from the traditional Chinese pharmacopeia—in *ramuan* preparations for men's health, while Malay bidan use *manjakani* oak galls (*Cympsgallae tinctoria)*, in promoting women's health. The use of such galls is believed to have originated in ancient Egypt and came to the Malay Peninsula via Arab traders or Unani physicians.

The Meaning of Ramuan

Malaysian culture represents a unique melting pot of knowledge and practices derived from Malay, Chinese, Indian and indigenous people's traditions. The multicultural and multi-ethnic diversity of the population means that Malaysia has inherited a unique confluence of different traditional medicine systems. Historically, the art of Malaysian healing and beauty is a manifestation of these influences. This traditional knowledge of health and beauty within such a multi-racial community has been practiced and enriched for generations.

In the old days, one would go no further than the garden and kitchen to clean the hair and body or even to get cures for common ailments. A whole plant or parts of plants (such as leaves, stems, barks, fruits, roots), and mixtures of plants and plants' parts are used and consumed. The therapeutic formulations produced from these mixed ingredients are called *ramuan*.

Generally, *ramu* or *ramuan* are defined as ingredients used in cooking, medicine, drink and food. Further definitions include:

:: *Ramu, Ramuan* (n)–ingredients, things, spices, seasoning
:: *Peramu* (n)–a collector; a person who looks for ingredients to formulate medicines
:: *Beramukan* (v)–to use ingredients
:: *Meramu* (v)–to look for ingredients needed to make something; to collect something
:: *Peramuan* (n)–research, study; products from ingredients

In the Malay classical language dictionary, *ber~ramu* means to collect or to look for leaves, fruits and roots for medicinal ingredients. In the old days, a practitioner or healer used to ask, '*Di mana ramu-ramu itu?*' (Where are the therapeutic ingredients?) when he or she wanted to prepare the mixtures for health or beauty concoctions.

Another term commonly used is *rempah ratus* (a term to denote a polyherbal preparation which requires a hundred kinds of medicinal plants and spices). And, in the villages, it is more common to find terms like *ramuan akar kayu* (plant roots mixture) and *ramuan asli* (original plants mixture).

In a broader context, the term *ramuan* encompasses the sense of ingredients blending together; it denotes a sense of 'melting pot', of unity and integration as well as the sense of 'many held together within unity'. *Ramuan* reflects the way of diversity within unity—a very Malaysian way.

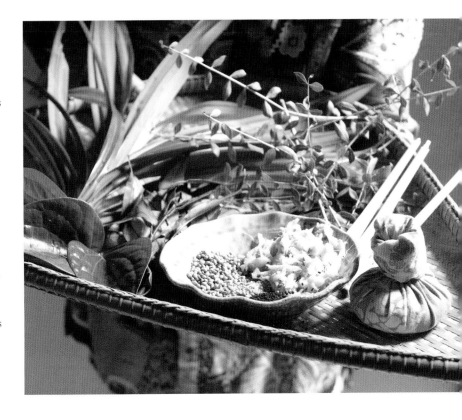

The Spice Route: Piquant Flavors in Food and Health

The Malay Peninsula has long been an important factor in the spice trade. Over two millennia ago, Indian and Chinese traders were shipping spices such as nutmeg, cloves, pepper and cinnamon from Kadaram—situated in the modern-day Malaysian state of Kedah—to West, South and East Asia. During the medieval era, as the Malay Peninsula was situated along the Asia to Europe trading routes, merchant ships regularly stopped off in ports such as Melaka to re-stock and trade. At this point, Arab traders dominated the trade. By the colonial era, the Portuguese, Dutch and British so prized these culinary spices, that the region became known as the Spice Islands.

Some spices were even used as currency, and because of the Malay Peninsula's geographical position, Malay became the language of regional trade. Naturally, these spices were used not only for food flavoring, but for

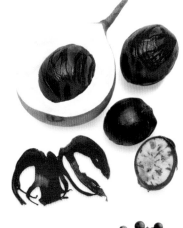

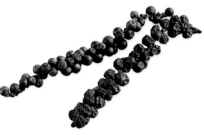

Top to bottom Nutmeg; black peppercorns; early trade routes and trade centers.

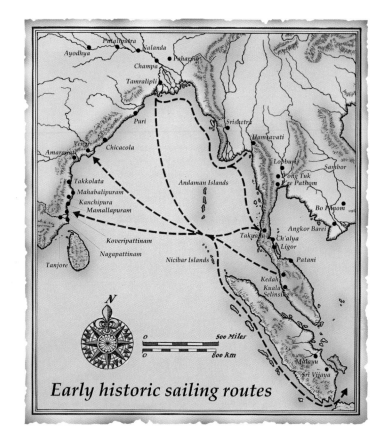

Early historic sailing routes

health benefits as well. As the more peppery spices caused sweating, they were associated with improving health and used as aphrodisiacs.

:: **Nutmeg** (*Myristica fragrans*) is known as *buah pala* in Malay and is the source of two spices, namely the nutmeg, the seed of the fruit, and mace, the lacy reddish arillus, or covering, on the seed. Both are widely used as food flavoring agents, while the essential oil, obtained by steam distillation of ground nutmeg,

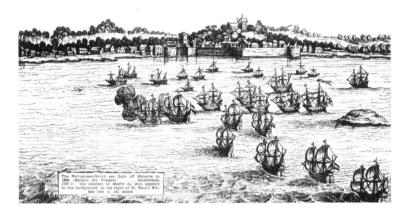

Malacca

The Portuguese–Dutch sea fight off Malacca in 1606 (Recueil des Voyages Amsterdam, 1701–7): the convent of Madre de Dios appears in the background, to the right of St. Paul's Hill. See text p. 181 below.

has high antioxidant properties and the essential oil extracted from its leaves has antimicrobial properties.

:: **Cloves** are another widely sought after commodity: known locally as *cengkih*, they are the dried flower buds of the tree *Syzygium aromaticum*. Traditionally, cloves are prescribed extensively as a painkiller in dental emergencies and as a remedy for stomach disorders and flatulence. Clove oil is also used to treat acne, pimples and other skin disorders.

is used in both the pharmaceutical and perfumery industries. Research indicates that nutmeg helps in reducing gastric acid secretion, cholesterol levels and in boosting libido levels.

:: **Black pepper** (*Piper nigrum L.*), known locally as *lada hitam*, is one of the oldest, most commonly used and most sought after spices worldwide. Called the 'King of Spices', its history dates back two millennia when it was first bartered between Melaka and China. Now, Malaysia is one of the major suppliers of black pepper to the world market. It is prescribed by various cultures for ailments such as constipation, diarrhea, indigestion, joint pain, liver problems, toothaches and tooth decay. Its spiciness is attributed to the presence of the chemical piperine, a substance that is believed to have antioxidant,

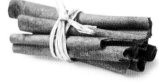

anti-inflammatory and anti-tumor potential. Black pepper is included in *ramuan* as one of the more important ingredients, particularly in formulations for men.

:: **Cinnamon** or *Cinnamomum verum* (from the Lauraceae family) is the bark of the cinnamon tree and has wide usage as a condiment and flavoring agent. Traditionally, it was prescribed for the treatment of colds, diarrhea and other problems related to the digestive system and was also used to treat bad breath. Known as *kayu manis*, it

Top to bottom A Portuguese–Dutch sea fight off Melaka in 1606. Wars were waged to gain monopoly of the spice trade; cinnamon sticks; dried cloves and flowers from the clove plant.

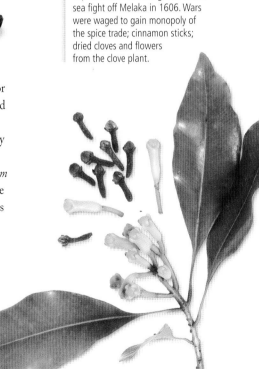

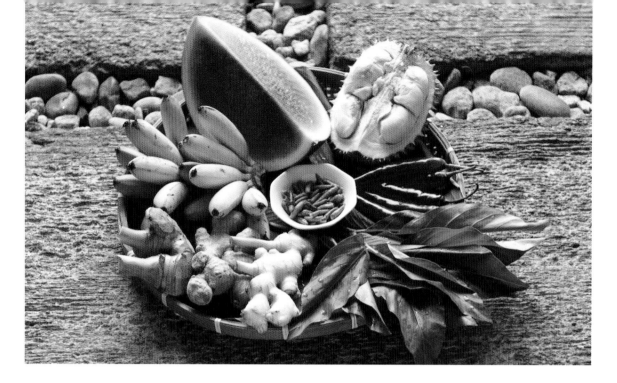

The Concept of Balance

The Malay belief that the universe—and humans within it—is composed of four major elements (earth, fire, air and water) is clearly akin to Ayurvedic and Chinese medical classifications. It is thought that if these elements exist and function in an orderly manner both within the body and in interaction with the social and physical environment, health is the result. An imbalance, conversely, leads to ill health.

Furthermore, Malay medicine postulates a humoral theory which stipulates that each individual is made up of four humors, the properties of which are hot and moist (blood), cold and moist (phlegm), hot and dry (black bile), and cold and dry (yellow bile). The theory advocates that each humor needs to be in perfect balance. If there is too much of one or not enough of another, remedies—in the form of herbs, incantations, diet, therapies and more—may be given.

Malay medicine also emphasizes the importance of maintaining an equilibrium of body temperature. Groups of foods are classified as having 'hot' or 'cold' properties. Acting individually or as a compound, they have an influence on a

Malays believe that if the four major elements (earth, fire, air and water) are in balance, health is the result.

Above A sampling of 'hot' foods.

Opposite 'Cold' foods include the starfruit and papaya.

Hot and Cold: Food, Medicine and the Body

In line with Malay humoral theory, Malay medicine postulates that most of the plants used in common healthcare can be categorized as 'hot', 'cold', 'moist', 'dry', 'windy' and/or 'gassy'. For example, such plants as *tongkat ali* (*Eurycoma longifolia*) and *sirih* or betel leaves (*Piper betle*) are considered 'hot and moist'; lemongrass (*Cymbopogon citratus*) is 'hot and dry'; long beans (*Vigna unguiculata* L.) are 'cold and windy'; and the much-loved durian (*Durio zibethinus*) is 'hot and gassy'.

Whether these items are taken as medicine or as food to promote general health is immaterial; similarly, they may be taken orally, used externally, or mixed together to form a typical *ramuan* preparation. What is important, however, is the combination of such foods.

For example, if certain plants, fruits, herbs or vegetables fall into the categories of 'hot and windy', 'hot and gassy', or 'cold and windy', they can only be consumed as food if the person does not suffer from an excess wind problem, water retention or migraines, or is not susceptible to chills. Furthermore, if that person has a hernia, a bone fracture, has joint, nerve or muscle spasms or pain, or is a mother in confinement, the consumption of such foods is not recommended. However, external usage for medicinal purposes is deemed safe.

Another example concerns the 'hot and gassy' durian. Malays believe that this prized fruit should not be consumed along with—or immediately after—any gassy drink. If a person were to be so foolhardy, the durian gas may explode in the stomach, causing pain, difficulty in breathing and even death. Another prohibited combination is the consumption of watermelon and milk at the same time. Watermelon falls into the categories of 'hot and moist', milk is considered 'cold and moist'. If the two are mixed together, it's thought that the milk will curdle, resulting in colic, indigestion, nausea, vomiting or diarrhea. Children who drink milk as part of a healthy daily diet are advised to steer clear of watermelon.

Certain traditional social practices reflect this categorization of foods. Malaysians often drink water that has been stored in a durian shell: this is not only because the durian is a highly beloved fruit, it is also because there is a health benefit involved. The Malays believe that the 'durian water' imparts a 'cooling' effect onto the body and hastens the expulsion of any heat and gas that may have been consumed earlier. As with many such practices, there is also a common-sense element that cannot be ignored.

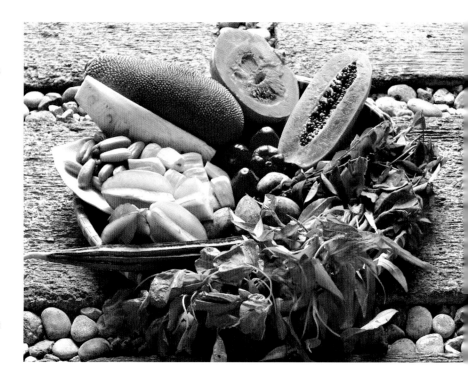

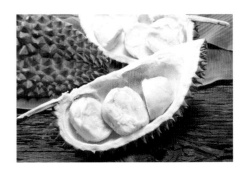

person's physical condition. The terms 'hot' and 'cold' are not specifically associated with temperature, but rather indicate the latent properties associated with particular dietary items. Thus, a sensation of coolness can be felt after eating mangosteen or cucumber. Similarly, a sensation of heat may be experienced after consuming spices such as red chili peppers or certain fruits such as durian. Indeed, mangosteen is commonly known as the fruit to eat after feasting on the 'hot', pungent durian. Mangosteen's sweet and cooling influence reduces the durian's fabled heat.

In addition, the Malaysian hot–cold theory of wellness includes such folk beliefs as *pantang larang* or prohibitions and taboos associated with observation and knowledge of the natural and spirit worlds. These were formulated to prevent the occurrence of disease, limit the severity of illness or restore wellbeing—and, in many cases, are pure common sense.

The hot–cold concept is not only found in the domain of food and medicine. Rather, it embraces the larger, holistic world view of the Malays. To a significant extent, Malay humoral beliefs permeate the physical, mental, emotional and spiritual worlds. In pregnancy, for example, coolness is associated with a healthy female state for conception to take place, while if the womb is excessively hot, a miscarriage may occur.

Concepts and Theories of Ill Health

Penyakit, the Malay term for illness or disease, indicates problems involving physical discomfort or lack of ease caused by either physical or mental disturbance or both. It may manifest itself in *lenguh* or aches and *sakit-sakit* or pains including fatigue, weakness, paleness, loss of appetite and heavy perspiration.

Above The durian, known as the king of fruits, is pungent and considered a 'hot' food.

Opposite, clockwise from top *Gaharu* fruits; gaharu wood chips; a gaharu tree.

Multiple Names, One Resin

Agarwood, aloeswood, *gaharu*, *karas*, *oudh*, eaglewood and *jinkoh* are only some of the names given to a fragrant resin produced by a fungal infection in trees of the genus *Aquilaria*. Since antiquity, gaharu has been used for traditional medicinal purposes and is still an important ingredient in Ayurvedic, Tibetan and East Asian medicine. It was highly valued in several cultures between South Asia and the Far East, and as early as the 3rd century BCE it was listed in the Chinese *Nan Zhou Yi Wu Zhi* with an

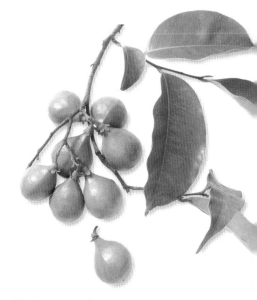

account of how native people collected it from the forests.

Greatly prized the world over for its usefulness in medicine, perfume and incense, the species is now seriously threatened. Because the resin is usually hidden deep within the center of only a few old trees, many trees have been indiscriminately felled over the centuries, so much so that there is serious concern as to the species' survival.

Native to Malaysia, Vietnam and Indonesia, there are five species of *Aquilaria* found in Malaysia: *A. malaccensis*, *A. microcarpa*, *A. hirta*, *A. rostrata* and *A. beccariana*. In 1995, *A. malaccensis* was listed by the Convention on International Trade in Endangered Species of Wild Fauna and Flora (CITES) as being endangered. This limits its export to only those trees obtained legally and harvested in a way that is not detrimental to the survival of the species. Currently, efforts are underway to cultivate *Aquilaria* and inoculate the trees chemically and organically to stimulate and enhance the production of the resinous hardwood.

So why is this wood so special?

Agarwood smoke and oil are highly prized as perfume in Asia and the Middle East. The oleoresin, obtained from steam distillation of the wood, is utilized in the production of the famous *attar* commonly used by

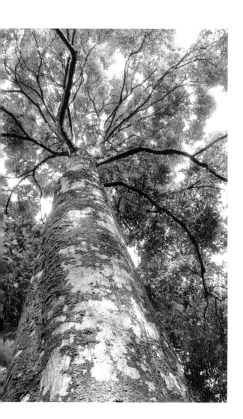

Muslims to give fragrance to prayer clothes. It is also used by Buddhist monks to deepen meditation, and has found its way into important Buddhist, Muslim and Hindu rituals and festivals.

In Malaysia, gaharu is valued for its appealing and distinctive fragrance and is mixed with coconut oil as a liniment to treat rheumatism and other aches and pains. It is also prescribed for jaundice, smallpox, abdominal complaints and in the treatment of dropsy, heart palpitations and as a tonic during pregnancy.

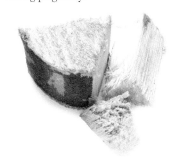

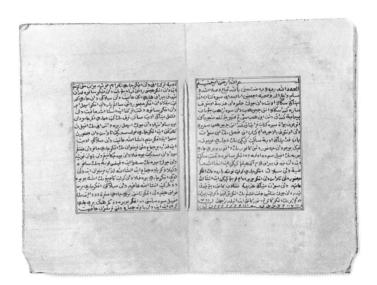

An old manuscript on traditional Malay medicine, written in 1872 CE, indicates that many febrile illnesses, vomiting, headaches, respiratory problems and ailments associated with the eyes, ears and nose have long been common among the general populace. For each category, appropriate herbal remedies were prescribed. A major category of illness cited in the treatise was *demam* or fever, which was generally considered to be caused either by *angin* (wind), *darah* (blood), *balgham* (mucus or phlegm) or *pitam* (a rush of blood to the head causing dizziness).

Cosmology also plays an important role in life, applying not only to the changing climate, but also pervading social, economic and religious matters. For example, when someone wants to build a house or start to plant rice, he should choose a date that corresponds with the rising moon. Healers also rely on cosmology. In making a diagnosis, they take into consideration which month the illness began; it is believed that this helps them to counter the cause of the problem more efficiently.

Blood or darah is a potential source of disease and illness. Though it is a vital element for growth, it should not be present in excess, or, it is believed, the body can become paralyzed.

Another important element in traditional diagnosis by the Malay bomoh is wind or angin. As a causative factor of illness, it can originate from outside the person, predisposing him or her to become *sejuk dan menggigil* or 'chilly and shivering', or it can dwell within the person. Angin circulates freely in the blood, and in excessive amounts can lead to the obstruction and clogging of the venous and arterial systems, thus preventing the body from maintaining a stable, healthy condition.

A body that has *banyak angin* or an 'excess of wind' is in a state of imbalance. Expelling this wind is a priority and may be achieved through massage and herbal formulations. In some cases, in a ritualistic trance performance, the shaman attempts to expel angin trapped in the body of a sick person.

Medicinal Plants and their Uses

Maintenance of good health and prevention of illness are emphasized in day-to-day life, with traditional healers advocating a diet that contains an essential balance of sweet, salty, sour and bitter elements. However, if remedies for illness are necessary, these are usually plant-based. Their basic purpose is to restore the chemical balance of 'heating' (*panas*) and 'cooling' (*sejuk*) elements within the body.

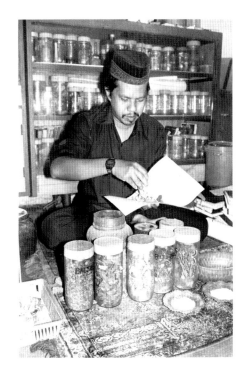

The selection of plants used in Malaysian herbal remedies depends on the combination of their medicinal properties. A combination of 40 or 44 different plants is traditionally considered most efficacious by healers, but the practice of combining plant ingredients in odd numbers—such as three, five or seven—also exists. What is most important in any combination of *ramuan*, however, is the inclusion of a plant called *ibu ubat* or 'mother of medicine'. This is a single plant believed to contain the essential healing properties required to affect a cure.

Bomoh may resort to using only an ibu ubat in times of emergency, but, in general, the combination should comprise more ingredients with a 'cooling' effect and less with 'heating' properties. Just as modern cancer treatment, for example, uses a principle of poly-pharmacy or multiple drugs in a single administration, so Malay medicine uses multiple ingredients in a single preparation for achieving different pharmacological effects. The overall aim is to restore generalized balance within the body's systems.

Herbal remedies incorporate various distinct plant parts including roots, rhizomes, barks, stems, fruits, flowers and seeds. Certain plants, particularly herbs, are generally consumed in their entirety as their known medicinal properties are not stored in one particular part. Remedies for *teruk* (serious or chronic) diseases normally require multiple treatments from a combination of plants. The effectiveness of these herbal remedies may be seen following regular use over a relatively long period. Over-consumption of any particular plant should be avoided.

Herbal ingredients are not only consumed for medicinal use, but are taken as part of daily meals. Most Malays are aware of the positive health effects of their traditional salad or *ulam* (see pages 98–102); such approaches to health maintenance and promotion are structured around a deep understanding of the properties of plants and the nature of illnesses. For example, red chilies (*Capsicum frutescens*), which belong to the 'hot and dry' category, are thought to be good for dispersing wind in the body, while *manjakani* galls, which belong to the 'cold and dry' category, are helpful for normalizing blood circulation, especially during menstruation.

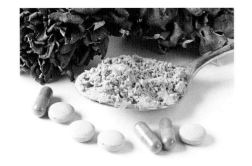

Below Pre-packaged herbal preparations make consumption more convenient.

Sambung Nyawa: The Hundred Ailments' Plant

Sambung nyawa (*right*) is the Malay name for *Gynura procumbens*, a small plant indigenous to Malaysia that is widely used in local traditional medicine. In Malay, sambung nyawa means 'prolongation of life'. Its much-vaunted general healing properties resonate as well in its Chinese name, *bai bing cao*, which translates as the 'one hundred ailments' plant'. The name is believed to be of Peranakan origin.

A vigorous climber in the Malaysian rainforest, the plant is now cultivated commercially and is found in many private gardens, *kampung* plots and even urban flower pots. Flowering cultivars of the species have also been developed and are now popular as house plants in temperate countries.

The leaves have long served in Malaysia as a flavoring for food. And as a medicine, the plant is used for kidney trouble, dysentery and as a febrifuge. Among its many pharmaceutical properties, it is considered anti-pyretic and anti-inflammatory. In traditional medicine, it is employed for a variety of ailments including migraine, constipation, hypertension and diabetes mellitus. It is deemed anti-carcinogenic and anti-allergic and the mashed dried leaf is often used as a salve for rashes. The leaves are also used in dermatological care and as a cosmetic skin elixir.

Now processed and marketed in capsule form, sambung nyawa is offered as a centuries-old cure from deep in the jungle for promoting general health and vitality. Specifically, it is held to be a potent aid for heart and cardiovascular conditions, for help in combating rheumatism and promoting blood sugar regulation, as an anti-viral and, as its name suggests, to prolong a healthy and productive life.

In addition, some herbal combinations are available as pre-packaged preparations in the form of pills, powders, ointments and tonics. Designed for both internal consumption and external applications, they are 'ready-made' versions of traditional formulae. Most are designed to expel excess wind from the body.

Chinese and Indian Malaysians, as well as Malays, commonly purchase these brand-name traditional medicine products, illustrating how integrated the Malay system is within society in general. In fact, whether the product is freshly made or out of a packet is irrelevant. Many Malaysians, from all walks of life and all ethnic groups, rely on these products for general wellbeing and health.

Certain plants, particularly herbs, are generally consumed in their entirety, as their known medicinal properties are not stored in one particular part.

The Betel Quid

Most Malaysians are well versed in the properties of common herbs and plants, so many will be familiar with the effects of the betel quid. The habit of chewing such quids (pellets) is widespread in Southeast Asia. Generally containing areca nut, slaked lime, gambier and sometimes clove wrapped in a betel leaf, the betel quid has long been part of Malay culture. Betel quids are chewed for many reasons, including for their stimulant effects, to satisfy hunger, to sweeten the breath, and as a social practice.

Nearly every Malay house, rich or poor, has a *tepak sirih* or betel quid box where the ingredients for the quid are stored. The Malays take great artistic pride in creating such boxes, utilizing different materials including wood, copper, silver and gold. Many are intricately designed and carved and some are embedded with pearls and gemstones. In many Malay meetings or gatherings, if the tepak sirih is not presented, it is a sign that the ceremony has been cancelled. If the betel quid box is taken away in the midst of a conversation or meeting, it signifies disapproval.

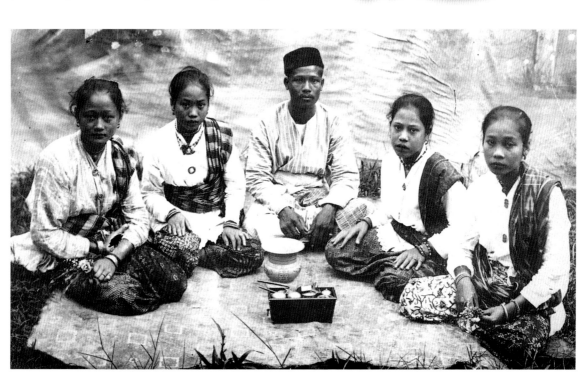

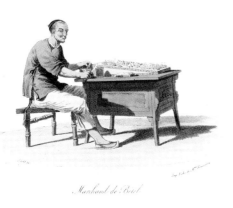

Marchand de Betel

In a marriage proposal, the tepak sirih takes center stage in the procession leading to the bride's house. In such cases, the ingredients include betel leaf, areca nut, slaked lime, gambier, cloves, tobacco and jasmine flowers. If the box is accepted, and small portions of each ingredient returned to the groom, it signifies that the bride's family accepts the proposal. If the marriage proposal is not welcome, the tepak sirih is returned untouched. This subtle system allows people to decline a proposal without causing outright embarrassment.

The Malays believe that the collective effect of the quid ingredients is anti-aging. In line with the 'hot–cold' theory of food, it's thought that the betel is initially warming, then becomes cold and dry; the *kapur* or slaked lime is warm; the *pinang* or areca nut is cold and temperate; and the *gambir* or gambier is cold and dry. When the ingredients are mixed together and chewed slowly, practitioners report increased awareness, a quickening of heartbeat and excess production of saliva. Somewhat habit-forming, the betel quid is part and parcel of the cultural fabric of Malaysia.

BETEL LEAF QUID INGREDIENTS

:: **Betel** (*Piper betle*) is the leaf of a vine belonging to the Piperaceae family, sometimes called the pepper family, which includes pepper and kava. It is valued as a mild stimulant, carminative and sialagogue (an agent that stimulates the flow of saliva). It has glossy, heart-shaped leaves, and grows profusely throughout the region.

:: **Betel nut** or **areca nut** is the seed of the fruit of the oriental palm *Areca catechu* and is also a stimulant. It can be intoxicating, producing giddiness in some people, and is also an astringent and a noted de-wormer.

:: **Gambier** (*Uncaria gambir*) may be best known for its usefulness in tanning and dyeing, but, when mixed with curcumin, gambier extract is used in skin whitening products for the treatment of age spots, freckles and dark blemishes. It contains many catechins, substances that are antioxidant in activity.

:: **Calcium hydroxide**, traditionally called slaked lime, is a chemical compound with the chemical formula $Ca(OH)_2$. Generally bought as a white powder and typically used in minute amounts, it is obtained when calcium oxide (quicklime) is mixed or 'slaked' with water. It is held to rid the body of toxins and bacteria.

:: **Cloves** (*Syzygium aromaticum*) with their antioxidant properties help to sweeten the breath. Traditionally, cloves are prescribed as a painkiller for dental emergencies and as a remedy for stomach disorders and flatulence.

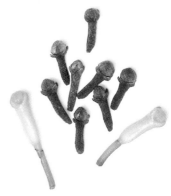

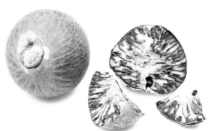

Opposite, top A traditional Malay *tepak sirih*, or betel quid box.

Opposite, bottom A Malay group in Sarawak in the early 1890s with a *tepak sirih*.

Clockwise from top A drawing of a Chinese betel seller, 1814; cloves help to sweeten breath; areca nuts.

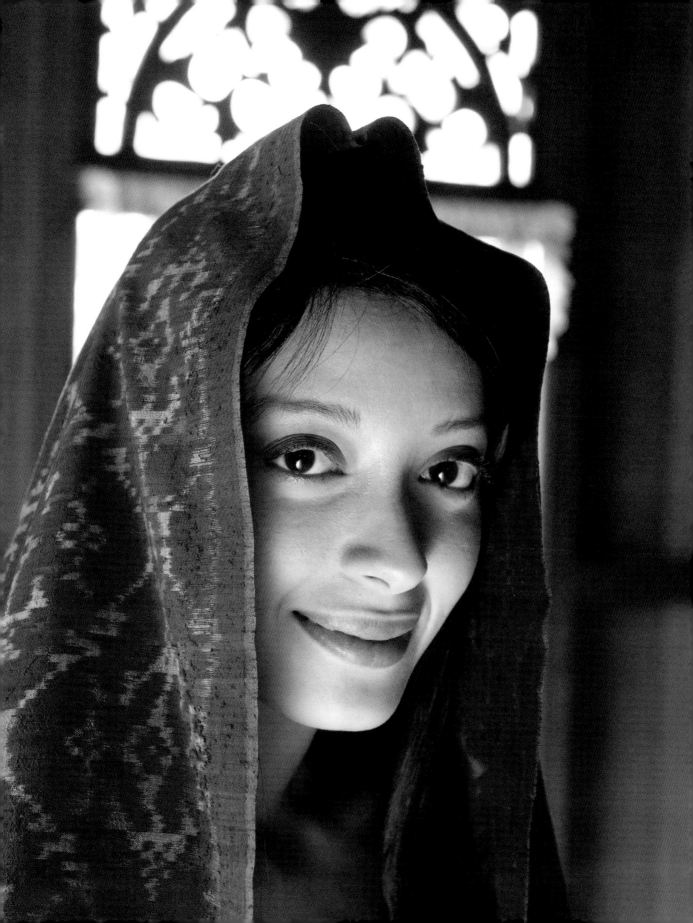

Discipline, Nature and Tradition
Malay Women's Health and Beauty

Malay women are esteemed, among other things, for their beauty, their courteous manners and their refined disposition and demeanor. Although the endearing elegance of Malay women is, to a large extent, the product of their social, cultural and religious backgrounds, other aspects of their beauty are grounded in a vast body of herbal healing knowledge that is passed down through the generations. As outer beauty is a reflection of inner health, the idea of inner and outer wellness as a totality is particularly prevalent in Malay culture.

In Malaysia, a shining complexion and bright eyes, as well as a cultivated restraint in manner, are particularly praised; Malay women are brought up to be mild-mannered, courteous and

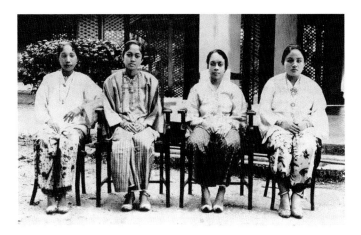

Opposite Malay women believe outer beauty is a reflection of inner health.

Right Malay women, c. 1930.

respectful towards their elders. That is not to say that they do not play an active role in public and private life. On the contrary, even before Independence in 1957, Malay women were actively involved in the public domain and, today, they are an economic and social force to be reckoned with. Women cabinet ministers, senior judges and CEOs of major corporations as well as the female governor of Malaysia's central bank all attest to the prominence of women in society. In the field of traditional Malay medicine, women commonly assume the roles of *bidan* (midwife), *dukun* (healer) and *pawang* (mystical specialist).

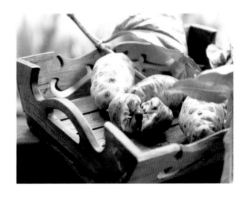

Above Noni fruits are used for hair care.

Below Special hair oil made of coconut milk, *keremak* leaves, *buah keras* and pandan leaves.

Opposite, above Ingredients in the warm herbal bath for teens include sweet lemongrass and slices of ginger.

Opposite, below Herbal tonic for teenage girls.

Health and Beauty Care

Traditionally, when a Malay girl starts to approach adulthood, she becomes the recipient of the wealth of herbal health knowledge that is stored, and sometimes documented, in the family. This knowledge comprises disciplines, rulings, remedies and traditions that have been handed down from generation to generation and includes some of the famed Malay anti-aging secrets. This pre-puberty period is a time of great excitement for the teenager, as she is finally gaining entrance into a world that was previously closed to her.

Pre-Puberty Rituals

Leading up to puberty, a number of specialized routines are introduced into most girls' lives. These include a weekly hair care regime, a twice-weekly massage and a purifying bath where crushed guava leaves (*Psidium guajava*) are used for cleansing. To this end, guava trees were commonly planted near traditional Malay bathing areas; leaves were literally plucked and used fresh as and when needed.

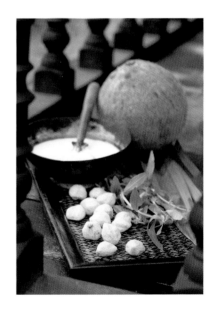

Blending fresh plants, fruits and herbs and applying them directly to the hair is a long-held Malay tradition: in a sequence that is natural, nutrient-rich and uplifting, mashed noni fruit (*Morinda citrifolia*) is applied to the hair and followed with a scalp massage using an oil of coconut milk (*Cocos nucifera*), *keremak* leaves (*Alternanthera sessilis* L.), *buah keras* (*Aleurites moluccana*) and pandan leaves (*Pandanus odorus*).

This hair and scalp treatment strengthens hair roots, promotes the growth of thick and glossy hair and gives the hair a wonderful aromatic scent. It is embedded in the conviction that early hair care delays premature graying of the hair later in life.

Feeding the skin, likewise, with body nutrients from nature helps stimulate blood circulation, and also moisturizes, softens and soothes the skin. Young teenagers are encouraged to apply a mixture of thick coconut milk and a pinch of salt all over the body to strengthen the skin, muscles and bones, all the while enhancing skin luster and shine.

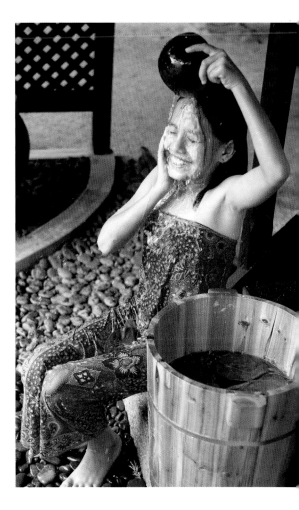

Puberty

When a girl reaches puberty, she is taught a number of other health and beauty rituals that relate to her developing body. Preventing period pains, strengthening the immune system and generally caring for her growing body are her priorities now. She may be given her first herbal tonic—a mix of sesame oil, egg yolk, pure honey and ginger juice—and be advised to keep away from cold baths, draughts and drinks.

The Malays believe that, during menstruation, the body is physically and spiritually weaker than during other times of the month, so prolonged exposure to cold temperatures is held to lead to low energy levels, anxiety and depression. In later life, these factors may lead to premature aging.

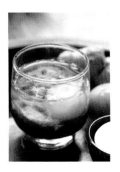

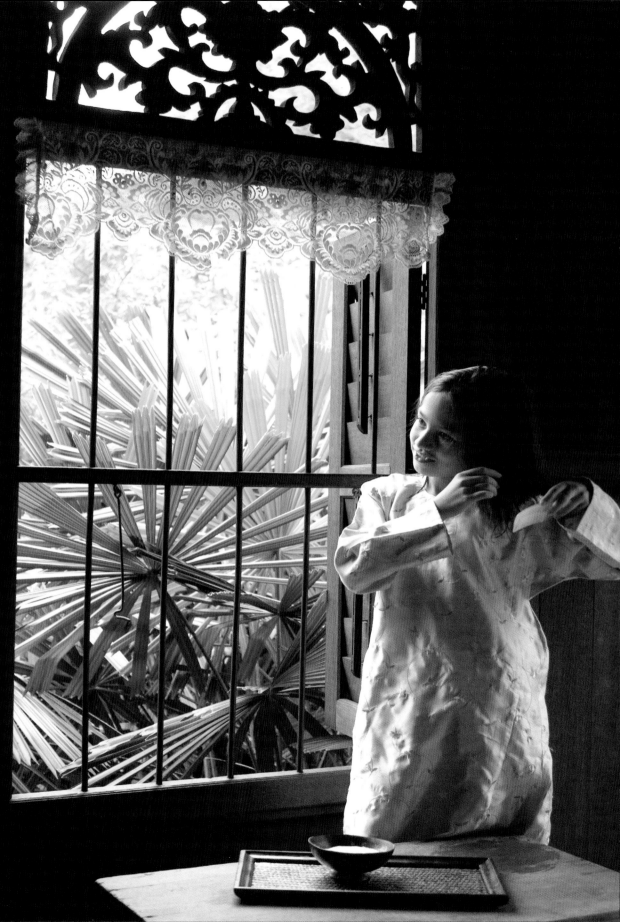

A warm herbal bath, therefore, is recommended. It often consists of sweet lemongrass (*Cymbopogan nardus*), betel leaves (*Piper betle*), pandan leaves and slices of ginger, all easily found in the compounds of the typical Malay house. The bath's aim is to ease out impurities and hot 'winds' by opening the body's pores: as the girl relaxes in this potent, enlivening mix, she is encouraged to let go of the old and welcome the new. Skin is invigorated and the immune system strengthened all the while.

Personal hygiene is also a top priority at puberty: an anti-fungal intimate washing formula that is both purifying and cleansing comes highly recommended. A mix of boiled henna leaves, betel leaves, *asam keping* (*Garcinia atroviridis*) and unprocessed salt, it eliminates odors, fights off infections and acts as a general deodorizer. Somehow, using such herbals makes bathing experiences more powerful, and knowing that they have been developed from centuries of tradition is all the more reassuring.

Facial Care

As with many other Eastern cultures, the Malays believe that the face is a reflection of the whole body. A fresh, radiant complexion indicates a well-balanced mind, body and spirit, while conditions such as dark circles under the eyes, puffiness, recurring blemishes, flakiness, dryness, oiliness and wrinkles reflect an imbalance somewhere within the wider body system.

The Malay belief system holds that water is the foundation of eternal youth, so it's a key ingredient in facial cleansing. Firstly, water is used to soften the skin and loosen dead surface cells, then, to enliven and refresh skin tone. Historically, Malay women washed with fresh coconut water or rice water, as opposed to

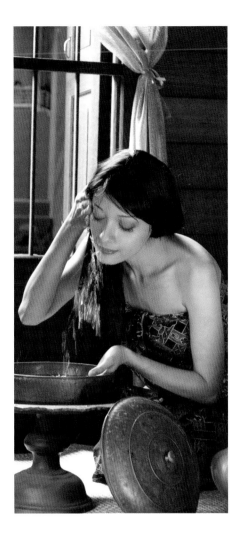

Opposite Traditionally, Malay teenage girls practice a number of specialized routines, such as a weekly hair care regime.

Above Malays believe water is the foundation of eternal youth and a key ingredient in facial cleansing.

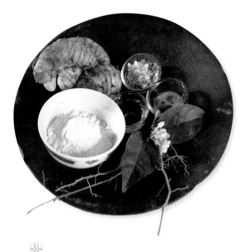

Above *Bedak sejuk*, or cooling powder, for Malay women.

Below *Ubat periuk* is considered a detoxifier and should be taken once a week.

Opposite *Lulut*, a scented body scrub made of turmeric and rice, is now an essential treatment offered at many Malaysian spas.

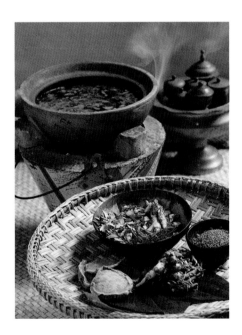

plain water, as they are thought to be more emollient and less drying for the complexion.

Then and now, Malay women use a special herbal powder known as *bedak sejuk*. Made from a powder of rice flour, jasmine roots and turmeric diluted with a little rose water, this soft paste is patted lightly onto face and neck. It helps to refresh the skin, resulting in a more supple and smooth complexion. Dry complexions use the powder diluted with coconut oil or olive oil, and, if applied alone, it is commonly known to help treat rashes, acne, pimples and pigmentation.

Skin Care

Changes to the skin occur throughout life and depend, in large part, on influences from the weather, seasons, growth phases, hormone levels, the condition of the body and mind, as well as the amount of tender loving care the skin regularly receives. An underlying belief in the Malay system holds that healthy, clear skin is directly attributable to a good blood flow with an equitable balance of acid and alkaline properties.

A once-a-week herbal brew, specifically geared towards skin health via internal cleansing, is *ubat periuk*. Among the ingredients used are senna leaves (*Cassia angustifolia*), betel leaves, galangal (*Languas galanga*), ginger (*Zingiber officinale*), *temu lawak* (*Curcuma xanthorrhiza*), *sepang* (*Caesalpinia sappan*), *jemuju* (*Carum copticum*), *cekur* (*Kaempferia galanga* Linn.) and *lempoyang* (*Zingiber aromaticum*). Drunk to overcome constipation, purge out heat and waste, remove fat and cleanse the blood, ubat periuk is a powerful detoxifier. Of course, this fits in with the Malay belief that internal cleanliness has direct outer consequences. The result of regularly imbibing this brew? A beautiful and youthful complexion, of course!

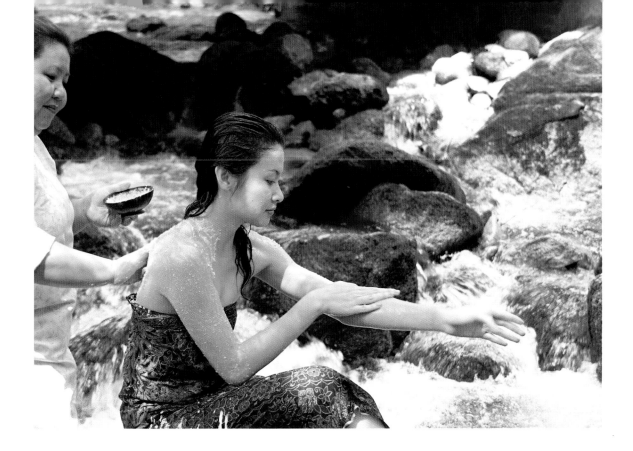

Another traditional skin care practice is a scented herbal scrub known as *lulut*. Now a staple on international spa menus, most popular lulut formulations use either glutinous or normal rice, cekur, sandalwood, ginger and *jerangau (Acorus calamus)*. Ground into a fine powder, it's mixed with a little rose water or pandan water to form a paste, then smoothed all over the body to exfoliate dead cells and promote new cell growth. The scrub's medicinal value is found in its anti-inflammatory and antioxidant properties; it also contains flavonoids, tannin and curcumin—all clear skin nutrients to boot.

Traditional Dental Care

Sweet breath, a strong, even set of teeth and healthy gums are another indication of health and beauty in the traditional Malay world. As such, dental care was facilitated with the use of areca nut shells *(Areca catechu)* burnt to an ash and rubbed onto gums and teeth; the addition of clove *(Eugenia aromatica*

Lulut has anti-inflammatory and antioxidant properties; it also contains flavonoids, tannin and curcumin—all clear skin nutrients to boot.

or *Syzygium aromaticum*) helped to strengthen gums and roots, prevent tooth decay and eliminate bad breath.

A quid of *sirih* or betel leaf, with a light touch of slaked lime, a pinch of gambier (*Uncaria gambir*), a thin slice of areca nut and a portion of a clove taken after a meal is a time-honored tradition among Malay women (and men as well) (see pages 40–41). A quid of betel leaf is also offered as a welcoming gesture when entertaining guests; many Malay houses have a *tepak sirih* or betel quid box where the betel leaves are stored. Many of these boxes are highly ornate made from carved wood, copper, silver or gold and may be studded with pearls and gemstones.

As with all such cultural practices, there's a health element involved. The quid doesn't just taste good after a meal, it's anti-aging too: betel leaf is an antiseptic that cleanses the blood and eliminates bad breath. Slaked lime helps in the process of breaking down stubborn fats and impurities, while gambier thins thick blood helping to avoid blood clots. Stress-relieving areca nut is known to strengthen teeth and gums; and cloves, with their aromatic and antioxidant properties, sweeten the breath.

Betel-chewing is a time-honored tradition among Malay women and men. A quid of betel leaf is also offered as a welcoming gesture when entertaining guests.

Malay Bridal Grooming

Andaman or bridal grooming is a very particular cultural practice, followed, to a lesser or greater degree, by many Malays. In the past, it sometimes lasted for a period of up to three months with a bride being confined indoors, preparing mentally and physically for her new life ahead. Today's andaman, however, has been distilled down to a few pampering-and-cleansing experiences given to a bride just before the marriage ceremony. Nevertheless, modern Malay brides follow in the footsteps of their ancestors' considerably stricter regimes.

Opposite Shaving of baby hair on the fringe of the bride's upper forehead.

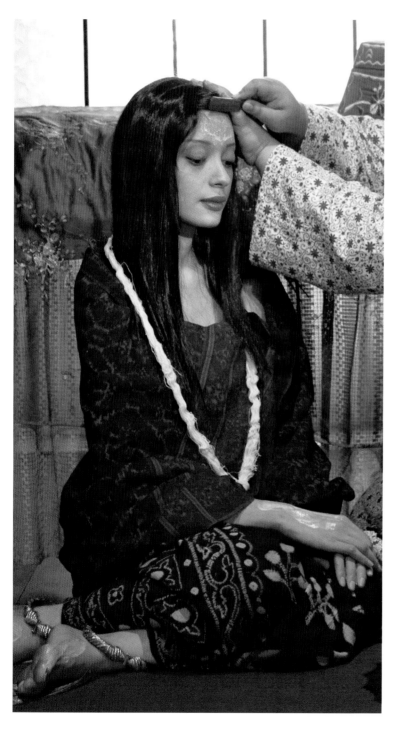

Ancient Rituals; Beautiful Brides

In ancient times, brides were allocated a *mak andam* or bridal attendant who was tasked with the responsibility of preparing the bride and bridegroom for their wedding ceremony. Her role (she was almost always a lady skilled in the arts of health and beauty enhancement) was to ensure that the couple participated in all the physical and spiritual rituals that were expected of them before the wedding ceremony took place.

The bride-to-be was given a special diet, a daily decoction of selected spices and herbs with aromatic properties, a daily bath, steam, hair scenting and oiling and plenty of advice and counseling. All these procedures, overseen by the mak andam, were designed to produce a 'true Malay bride': one with alluring, radiant health and beauty.

A Malay wedding is highly renowned for its pomp and pageantry. Usually spread out over several days, it starts with some preliminary beauty ceremonies followed by the *nikah* ceremony (the religious element), and culminates with the *bersanding* (the customary wedding during which the bride and groom sit close together).

In the old days, three days before the nuptial ceremony, the mak andam performed a private ritual known as *buang cangrai* or 'casting away of ill luck'. Taking a tray containing a young coconut, cut open and with the

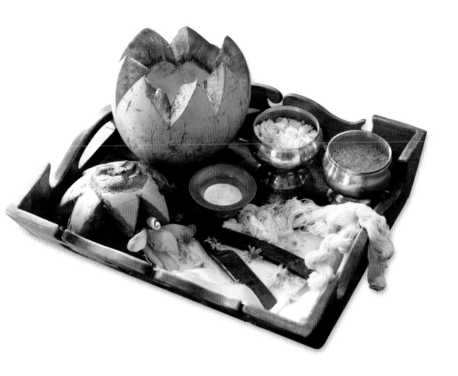

water still intact, a bowl of powder made from rice flour softened into a soft paste with rose water, a bowl of yellow rice (rice mixed with turmeric), a bowl of *bertih* (glutinous rice fried in the husk), a roll of *benang mentah* (unprocessed thread), a piece of white cloth and a shaving knife, she would begin the ceremony.

The bride sat neatly in the *bertimpuh* stance—a polite sitting posture in Malay culture—with her head covered. After a special welcoming prayer, the bridal attendant showered the bride with the yellow rice and bertih, then wiped her face with the coconut water, garlanded her hair with the unprocessed thread and poured water onto areas of the bride that were to be shaved.

Eyebrows were then plucked and shaped, any facial hairs removed through a process known as 'threading'

Traditionally, Malays believe that a spiritual betel quid helps to overcome anxiety, fear and stress, as well as enhance the aura (*seri*) of the bride. A bride's glowing beauty or aura is supposed to last up to 40 days, so the quid plays just a small part in supplying her with seri.

whereby unwanted hairs were extracted by rolling an unprocessed thread dipped in wax to pull hair out from the roots, and the treated areas covered with a soft herbal paste made of cinnamon, nutmeg, *pegaga* and white turmeric. This herbal paste had emollient properties and helped reduce any redness or

soreness induced by the plucking. Then came the shaving of *anak rambut* (the baby hair on the fringe of the upper forehead).

Two days before the nuptial ceremony, in the morning, the bride was given an 'aural enhancement bath' or *upacara naik seri*. Blessed floral water was poured from an earthen jug (see page 54) over the bride in a ritual purification ceremony; this was followed in the evening with the henna application ceremony or *berinai*. This was largely a family affair, with the grandmother, mother, sisters and close family members applying henna paste onto the fingers and toes of the bride in elaborate and beautiful patterns. Believed to ward away evil spirits and keep the bride healthy, henna application is, on a practical note, also helpful in preventing nail infections.

Finally, on the eve of the marriage ceremony itself, the mak andam

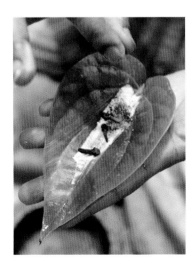

prepared the 'spirit of the betel leaf' or *sirih semangat* ceremony. The betel quid plays a significant role in Malay culture, so it is no surprise that it has a part in the wedding ceremony. Three quids—with a blessed betel leaf filled with gambier, slaked lime and clove— are carefully folded, then eaten at three key moments: the first at the religious solemnization of the marriage, the second the next day while the bride is being made up for the bersanding ceremony, and the third just before the bride joins the groom at the

ceremony. This is when she sits with her future husband together on the bridal couch before being escorted back to his house.

Traditionally, Malays believe that a spiritual betel quid helps to overcome anxiety, fear and stress, as well as enhance the aura (*seri*) of the bride. A bride's glowing beauty or aura is supposed to last up to 40 days, so the quid plays just a small part in supplying her with seri. As the three-day ceremony is an elaborate affair, with the bride treated as a queen

and her groom as a king, she needs to radiate beauty, poise and charm. Naturally, her radiance isn't superficial; rather, it is the culmination of her 100 days of preparation.

Opposite, above A tray of various items used in the *buang cangrai*, or 'casting away of ill luck' ceremony.

Opposite, below The *sirih semangat* is prepared on the eve of the marriage ceremony.

Below The henna application ceremony or *berinai*, largely a family affair, takes places two nights before the nuptial ceremony.

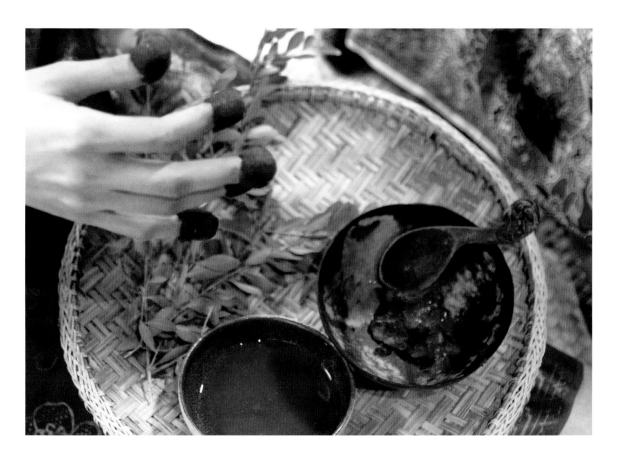

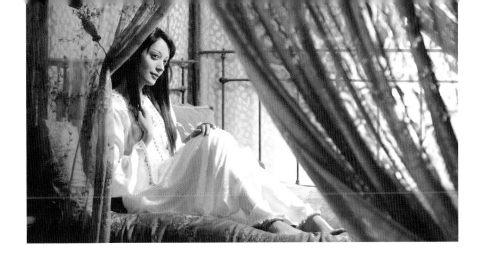

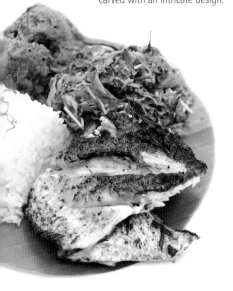

Traditionally, brides were supposed to remain closeted and out of sight, all the while following a special program of diet, herbs, baths and more. This program was designed to cleanse, refresh and rejuvenate. Foods were composed of dishes that contained only nutritional, fresh or dry-fried ingredients, all selected to optimize hygiene and health. Certain vegetables and soupy foods were not encouraged because they were considered to have *sejuk* or *angin* ('cold' and 'wind') values, and could result in the expelling of fluid, something that was not desirable. Similarly, the bride was given a daily decoction that was designed to induce sweet-smelling perspiration.

For skin and body care, the bride received a daily therapeutic floral bath that included a floral body scrub, floral hair wash, and scented sauna using exotic flowers such as roses, jasmine, two types of *cempaka* (*Michelia champaca* and *Michelia alba*), *kenanga* (*Cananga odorata*) and medicinal-aromatic woods such as sandalwood and *gaharu* (*Aquilaria malaccensis*). As the bride's body was scrubbed and scented, a sweet aroma permeated the room and refreshed the whole home. This was further intensified when the bride-to-be was showered with a specially brewed water of *seribu bunga* or 'thousand flower essence' using a coconut shell ladle scraped clean and carved with an intricate design.

Another body treatment consisted of herbal steaming. Specially formulated to provoke intense sweating, thereby eliminating toxins from the body, it is one of the quickest ways

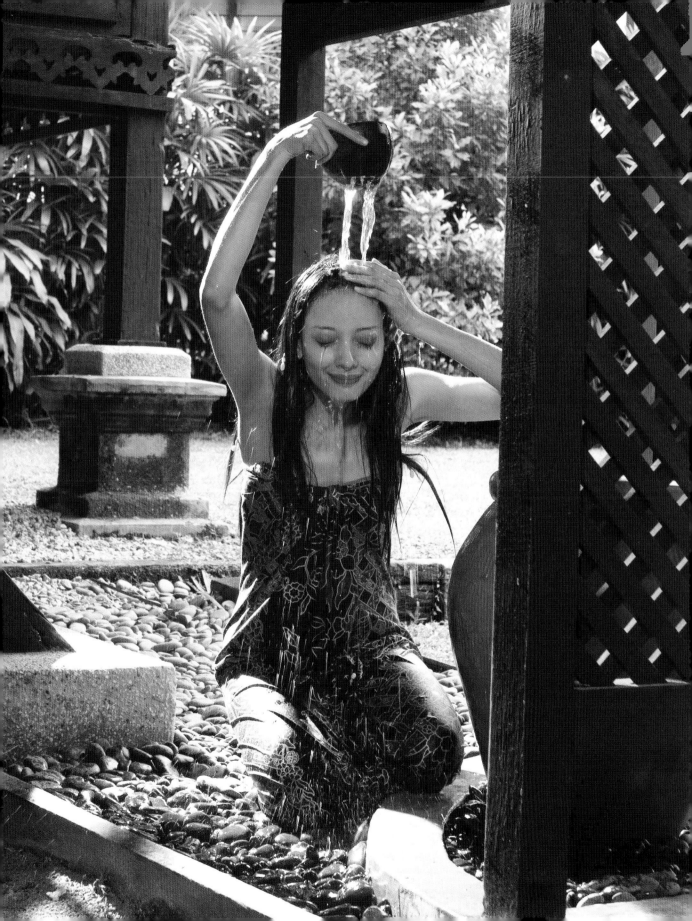

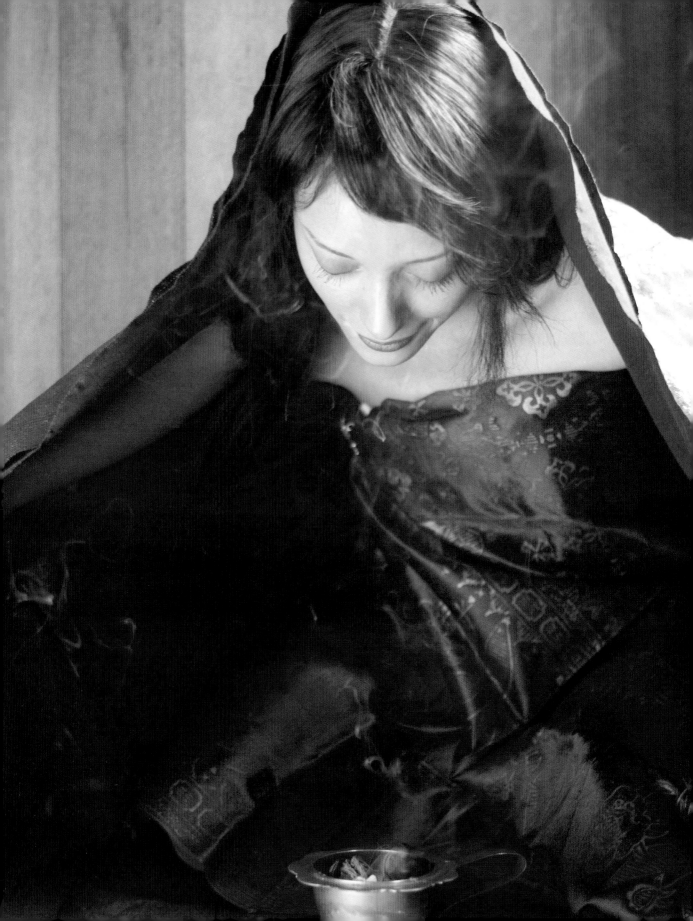

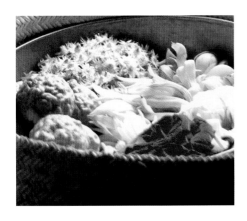

of bringing the body back to equilibrium. First the bride was rubbed all over with an oil made from the essence of *bunga tanjung* (*Mimusops elengi*). Then, as the floral ointment seeped through the body's pores, she sat over an earthenware pot or *buyung* filled with an aromatic concoction of boiling roots, flowers and rose water. The mouth of the pot was covered with a banana leaf, perforated with holes through which steam passed. Covered in a sarong, her body captured the properties from the herbs as she sweated. Toxins were eliminated and her body was cleansed. The finale to this was the drinking of an aromatic herbal concoction made with Kaffir lime and scented flower buds. It had a splendid scented effect on the whole body.

Aromatic hair steaming and scenting also has its roots in bridal preparations. This consists of passing a container smoking with gaharu charcoal and frankincense in and around the hair in order to leave a hauntingly sweet and lingering scent on skull and tresses. It's yet another example of how the bride is beautifully coiffed, pampered, scented and generally prepared for the most important day—and night—of her life. Today, many of these time-honored rituals have found their way into Malay spas (see pages 177–195).

Opposite Aromatic hair steaming.

Above A concoction of roots and flowers prepared by the bridal attendant.

Below Censer containing frankincense and *gaharu*, used to scent and steam the bride's body and hair.

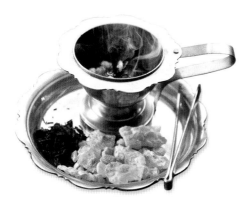

Malay Secrets of Anti-Aging

Unquestionably, everybody ages with time and has to come to terms with his or her own mortality. However, in the Malay tradition, a woman is encouraged to age with grace—and certainly not prematurely. After marriage, she is expected to follow a life-long maintenance program: designed to keep her looks youthful, her body supple, her skin firm, hair healthy

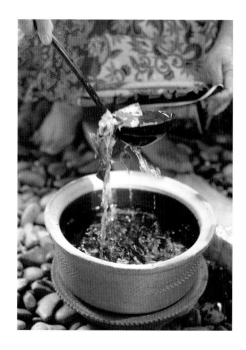

and her complexion radiant. The program covers all of the stages she experiences after marriage—pregnancy, childbirth, menopause and old age.

Kacip fatimah (*Labisia pumila*) and *akar serapat* (*Parameria polyneura*) are undoubtedly two of the most powerful tools a Malay woman has at her disposal. Used for centuries to firm up vaginal muscles and strengthen the uterus and cervix, when mixed with the betel quid combination of a tiny amount of slaked lime, areca nut, gambier and clove, kacip fatimah and akar serapat help with the general health of the vagina.

Another treatment, for the same purpose, is the herbal sitz bath. Customarily given once a day for three or seven days after a woman's period, this bath includes salt, *manjakani* (*Cympsgallae tinctoria*), betel and henna leaves, *mengkunyit* (*Coscinium blumeanum*), black seeds (*Nigella sativa*) and tamarind (*Tamarindus indica*). All these potent herbs are boiled and added to water in a small hip bath for personal hygiene and the maintenance of healthy vaginal tissues and muscles.

A dry herbal sauna called *tangas kering* is another traditional ritual formulated for cervical health, incontinence and an enlarged uterus. In times past, it wasn't uncommon to see a group of women sitting together chewing betel with kacip fatimah and akar serapat, chatting and passing the time. What the casual observer wouldn't have noticed, however, is that they each had a coconut shell containing a small round heated pebble on which was placed such pounded herbs as turmeric, Kaffir lime and *akar semalu* (*Mimosa pudica*) beneath their sarongs. As they relaxed together, they would actually be benefiting from this very particular type of feminine sauna at the same time!

Above The herbal sitz bath comprises salt, black seed and tamarind, among other ingredients.

Opposite, above Ingredients used for *tangas kering*, or dry herbal sauna.

Opposite, below Ingredients used to make *mantah wangi*, or floral elixir.

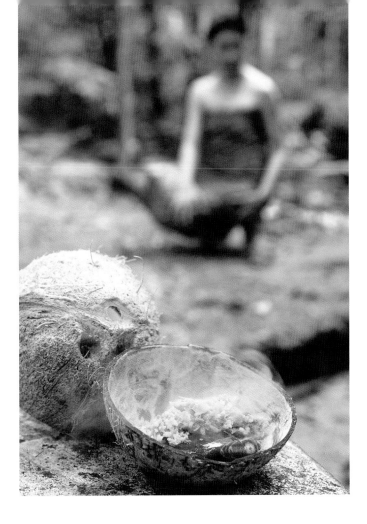

One of the most treasured and best-kept secrets of anti-aging in the Malay world is the *mantah wangi* or floral elixir. A known antioxidant, astringent, anti-inflammatory and carminative, it is unfortunately falling out of popular use today. However, it's an excellent way for women to balance their hormones. Made from the freshly ground flower buds of red roses, jasmine, bunga tanjung (*Mimusops elengi*), *senduduk putih* (*Melastoma imbricatum*), manjakani and *temu kunci* (*Gastrochilus panduratum*) and mixed with salt, it is stored in a banana leaf. When taken each morning, before breakfast, with warm water or pure honey, it's believed to firm and tighten skin and muscles, both internally and on the surface. As the Malays say, the inner mirrors the outer; internal health gives rise to an external glow.

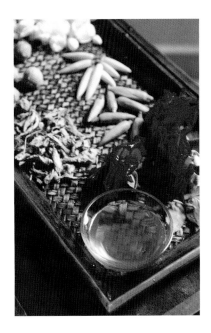

Below A special herbal massage oil
for pregnant women comprises coconut
oil, betel leaf, lemongrass, nutmeg, red
ginger and fenugreek.

Opposite A woman goes through
mental, emotional as well as physical
changes during pregnancy.

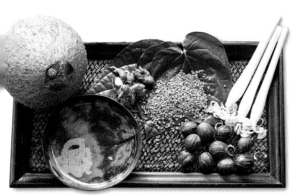

Pregnancy, Birth and Post-Natal Health

Many people comment on Malay women's slim figures and
erect postures, which many retain in spite of often bearing
many children. Exactly how these women manage their
pre- and post-pregnancy health is usually kept under wraps
within individual families, but most know that herbal remedies,
age-old practices and plant decoctions are important aspects
of the regime.

Unfortunately, because most of these practices are
undocumented and many women are now turning away from
what they consider the old 'folk wisdom' of their mothers and
grandmothers, this ancient knowledge is in danger of being
lost. Asian mothers are eschewing the old ways for newer,
Western science and technology with their instant fixes of
surgery, plastic or otherwise.

If a woman opts for a painless, speedy recovery, her outer
shell may shine, but there could very well be inner damage.
Prevention is far better than a cure. Traditional Malay herbalists
argue that the age-old methods, when practiced in the proper
context with patience and understanding, give long-term
benefits—both inside and out.

Pre-Natal Care

Pregnancy is a period of great physical and emotional
change for a woman, so it's natural that there are a number of
recommendations for the Malay pregnant woman. Her diet
is of the utmost importance, as is the self-care that she needs
to employ during all three trimesters. As mothers-to-be often
suffer from nausea and stress and strain on muscles and joints,
the Malay pharmacopeia is called upon to help her safely and
comfortably through pregnancy.

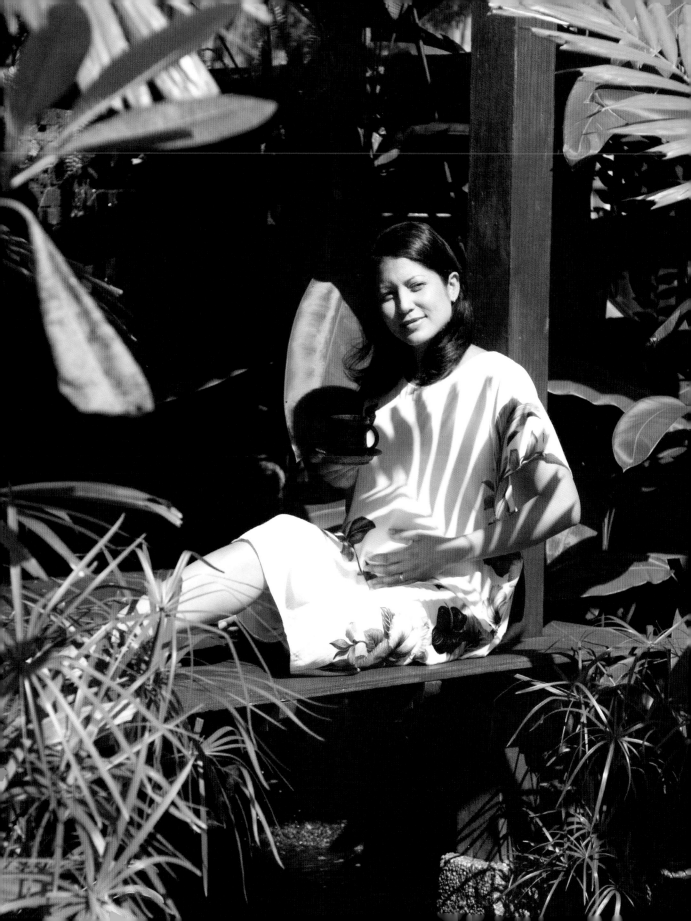

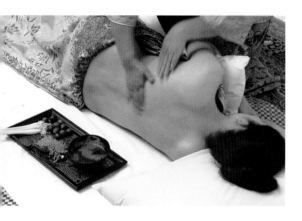

One popular remedy is massage, a soothing and beneficial therapy given only after the first trimester. Traditionally, in pre-natal massage, a traditional midwife or *bidan* applies only a special herbal oil of coconut oil, betel leaf, lemongrass, nutmeg, red ginger and fenugreek, but essential oil massages are fast gaining popularity these days. Appropriate essential oils can reduce stretch marks and de-stress pregnant women; soft effleurage of upward strokes on both legs and thighs boosts the circulation, relieves, prevents and reduces puffy ankles, and helps with varicose veins.

As the pregnancy progresses, the bidan performs a gentle massage with soft circular motions on the abdomen and pelvic area. This soporific movement helps to position the baby and brings relief to the pelvic muscles of the pregnant woman.

Post-Natal Care

In Malay society, a new mother traditionally returns to her mother's house to undergo a regimen of post-natal care with the help of her mother. She normally observes what is called a confinement period of 44 days. However, most women nowadays prefer to recuperate in their own homes with the help of a bidan.

Traditional post-natal confinement gives the mother a chance to rest and recuperate after the trauma of pregnancy and delivery. It helps the mother in many ways: physically, as the body is usually raw and tender after the strenuous exertion of labor; emotionally, as the new mother is adjusting to the challenges of motherhood and the arrival of a new family member; and mentally, as she rests and recuperates.

A healthy diet is of the utmost importance. Plenty of herbal salads, steamed chicken (the stock of which is believed to help

Above Massage is given only after the first trimester.

Below A sample of prohibited foods for mothers in confinement. It includes brinjal, pumpkin, bamboo shoots and legumes.

Opposite, above *Urutan sentuhan* starts from the feet and gradually moves up the legs with upward strokes to the upper thighs.

Opposite, below Medicated oil for perineum tears. It is made of *manjakani*, turmeric, nutmeg and coconut oil.

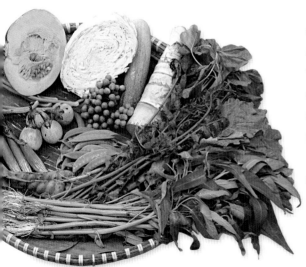

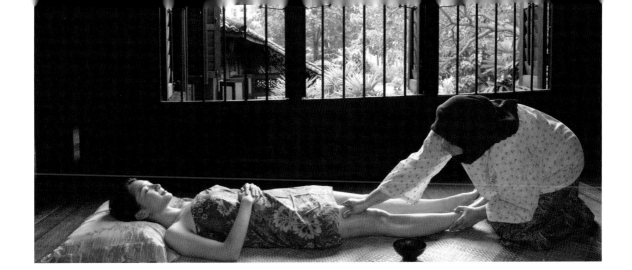

the body recover strength and resilience) and certain herbal decoctions are the order of the day. Seafood and particular vegetables and fruits with so-called 'cold' and 'wind' properties are discouraged, as are cold water, gassy drinks and fruit juices.

In addition to eating well, women are advised to rest as much as possible, as the treatment regime starts from the first day of delivery and is fairly intense. The first step has the bidan attending to any perineum tears with a medicated oil of manjakani, turmeric, nutmeg and coconut oil; this is antiseptic, anti-inflammatory, anti-bacterial, anti-fungal and emollient, so it hastens healing quickly and efficiently.

The early days also include a type of wellness massage known as *urutan sentuhan*. Lasting about 15 to 20 minutes, it starts from the feet and gradually moves up the legs with upward strokes to the upper thighs. The abdomen and lower back are also attended to, and, finally, the bidan massages the hands, shoulders, neck and face before finishing with a head and scalp massage. An anti-stress treatment, the massage's purpose is to relieve stomach cramps, loosen tense muscles and overcome fatigue. Using a medicated herbal oil, it helps the mother get a good night's rest, relaxing her and facilitating internal healing.

A few days later, a post-natal hot stone massage known as *urutan tuaman batu* is performed. Generally given from the fourth day after birth for 35 days, it is an ancient craft performed

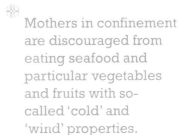

Mothers in confinement are discouraged from eating seafood and particular vegetables and fruits with so-called 'cold' and 'wind' properties.

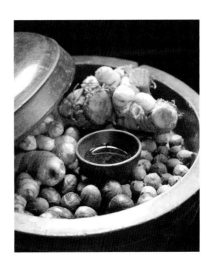

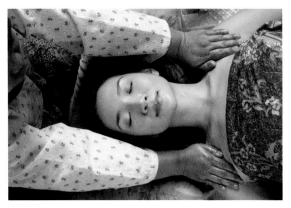
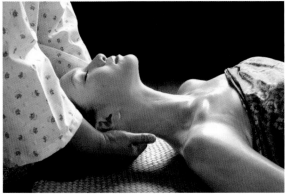

early in the morning just after the mother has consumed her first herbal tonic. Designed to relieve tense muscles, break down stubborn fats and eliminate trapped winds and toxins, this massage hastens the shrinkage of the enlarged uterus, flattens the abdomen and trims the body back to its pre-pregnancy figure. If this sounds truly wonderful, it's worth a try, as it is also immensely nurturing and relaxing.

Heated stones, traditionally made from seven layers of clay burned into a round shape, are laid on several layers of herbal leaves such as noni leaves, betel leaves, *bunga tahi ayam* leaves (*Lantana aculeate* or *Lantana camara*) and *daun lengkuas*

Clockwise from top left Shoulder massage, part of *urutan sentuhan*; one of the last few steps of the urutan sentuhan involves a head massage; *urutan tuaman batu*, or hot stone massage, is performed four days after giving birth; heated stones are laid on layers of herbal leaves.

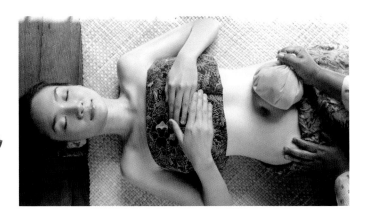

(*Languas galanga*), then bound in a cotton or *batik* cloth and rubbed all over the body. The bidan applies extra force and pressure on flabby and tense areas. As the heat seeps through the cloth, it transports the healing properties of the leaves deep into the tissues. Bliss!

In the third week, another type of massage, known as *urutan asak*, is introduced. This massage is designed to gently help the uterus 'find its way home', ease out any postpartum discharge and encourage the elimination of any stubborn impurities. It involves massaging the side of the pelvic area, not directly on the uterus or the cervical mouth area, and can only be performed by an experienced bidan.

This is followed by the final massage, *urutan sengkak*, a full-body massage that works on re-positioning the uterus. Also highly specialized, it should not be given if the uterus is still enlarged. A well-trained bidan knows when to commence urutan sengkak as Malay practice is very clear that forced massage on the uterus is strictly forbidden. Every massage type, in fact, should be performed in a patient manner— with a tender touch, in a firm yet caring manner, and only according to strict procedure. All massages, with the exception of urutan sentuhan, end with stretching movements aided by the masseuse.

During this time, a number of complementary treatments are performed to assist with the general aims of the various massages. The best-known is probably that of body binding or *bengkung* or *barut* in Malay. Designed to restrict overeating and to prevent entry of cold 'wind' via the abdominal pores, body binding also aids in the elimination of what Malays call 'hot and toxic air'. Its aim is to trim back the new mother's body and stomach, making it flat and firm without any stretch marks.

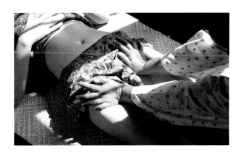

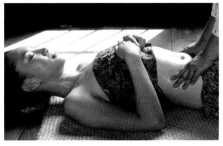

Top By massaging the side of the pelvic area in *urutan asak*, the midwife helps the new mother ease out postpartum discharge and eliminate impurities.

Above *Urutan sengkak* aims to reposition the uterus and should only be performed by a well-trained *bidan*.

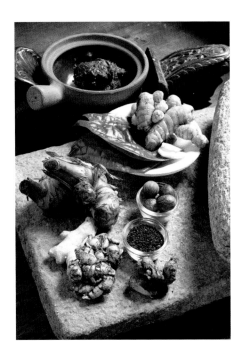

Above Ingredients that make up the *ubat barut*, applied all over the mother's abdomen during body binding.

Below Herbal pouch to relieve symptoms of agalactia, blockage in milk flow.

Opposite Body binding aims to trim the new mother's body and stomach.

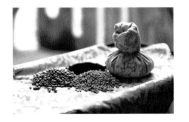

If this sounds too good to be true, it needs to be stressed that it isn't exactly the most comfortable practice in the world as the binding reaches from just below the breasts to down below the buttocks. The binding should be kept on for 23 hours of the day and is recommended for periods of 30, 44 or 100 days. Nevertheless, centuries of usage have seen it garner results—and many modern Malaysian women (Malay and non-Malay) swear by its efficacy.

Before the bidan wraps the body, she applies a medicated ointment called *ubat barut* all over the abdomen. There are many different types (and each bidan will undoubtedly proclaim the potency of her own particular recipe), but the best contain tamarind juice, betel leaf, black seed, turmeric, nutmeg, galangal and various other gingers including lempoyang, red and white ginger. The ointment encourages the contraction of the uterus, the breaking down of fats and cellulite in cells, and the reduction of multiple stretch marks, while the binding re-shapes the outer contours of the body.

The one hour out of the 24 when the mother is not bound up tight is used for herbal sitz baths, feminine saunas, post-natal body scrubs and other herbal baths that may be prescribed for particular ailments. For example, there's a special herbal pouch to help ease the flow of a mother's milk and another that helps with water retention or puffiness. With an experienced bidan, the mother is alternately bullied and berated, or cared for and cosseted, as, all the while, her body is coaxed back into its pre-pregnancy shape.

If this sounds hard, it can be. Yet, on the other hand, the post-natal period is full of intense new experiences, especially for first-time mothers, so being in the hands of an expert gives reassurance, calm and a common purpose.

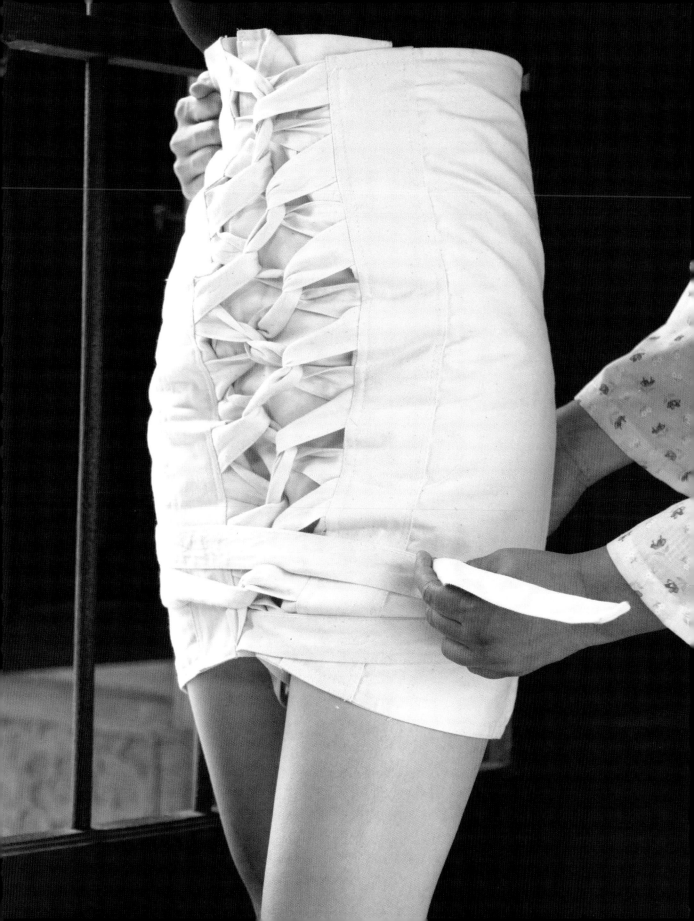

Specialist Herbs for Postpartum Remedies

The global interest in natural remedies is revitalizing local herbal industries in many parts of the world. In Malaysia, new technologies and a focus on preserving plants with medicinal value have resulted in increased manufacture of herbal preparations along with testing and clinical trials. Both are to be encouraged.

In the case of plants traditionally used as aphrodisiacs, for genital care and in postpartum recovery, the science is encouraging. Recent studies conducted by a research institute in Malaysia suggest *kacip fatimah* (*Labisia pumila, below*), for example, encourages the production of increased free testosterone from the ovaries. Kacip fatimah is also known to contain phytoestrogens and isoflavones and studies on the ethanolic extract of the root have shown that it exhibited weak, but specific, estrogenic effects, on cells. For women, whose estrogen supply drops substantially at menopause, this could be good news.

Kacip fatimah is lauded as a miracle wonder plant by local women. It is used for a variety of health benefits, from alleviating fatigue to firming abdominal muscles.

Thus, a plant that has been used by rural mothers and *bidan* for centuries, has not only received modern validation, but is also beginning to find its way into international markets—a promising trend.

So what are these particular herbs for postpartum remedies? And how can they help women around the world?

Kacip fatimah is probably the best known. Lauded as a miracle wonder plant by local women, it is used for a variety of health benefits: to contract the uterus after childbirth; to firm and tone abdominal muscles and tighten vaginal skin and walls; to ameliorate painful or difficult menstruation, cramping and irregular periods; and to alleviate fatigue and promote emotional wellbeing. It is also taken on a regular basis as a vitality, libido and energy booster.

Traditionally, fresh or dried kacip fatimah is boiled in an earthen cooking pot and the concoctions or decoctions taken on a regular basis with other herbs. Currently, kacip fatimah formulations are available in powdered or extract forms in pills, capsules, tea or coffee mixtures and even as a canned drink for ease of consumption.

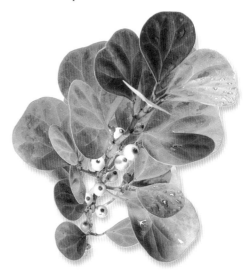

Mistletoe fig (*Ficus deltoidea, above*), known locally as *mas cotek*, is an epiphyte plant in the Moraceae family. Traditionally used as a postpartum treatment to help in contracting the muscles of the uterus and in the healing of the uterus and vaginal canal, it is also used as a libido booster by both men and women. Due to cross pollination, various forms, types and varieties of this *Ficus* (or fig) are found in the country. Normally, leaves and plant parts from various types and varieties of the species are mixed together to produce a potent blend.

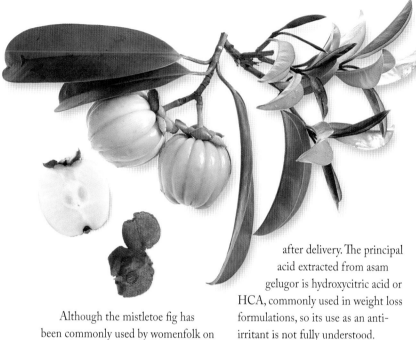

Although the mistletoe fig has been commonly used by womenfolk on the east coast of Peninsular Malaysia and in Sabah for centuries, it has not received much attention until recently. However, recent chemical analysis of extracts of mistletoe fig leaves from the various types has revealed different levels of active compounds, including bioflavonoids, tannins, phenols and triterpenoids—all of which contain antioxidant, anti-inflammatory, antiseptic and expectorant properties. As such, its prominence is expected to grow.

Less prominent, but useful as a soothing vaginal douche when combined with betel leaves, is a decoction of *asam gelugor* (*Garcinia atroviridis, above*). Frequently mixed also with such ingredients as turmeric, oak galls, guava leaves and mimosa leaves, it is helpful in clearing up vaginal discharges after delivery. The principal acid extracted from asam gelugor is hydroxycitric acid or HCA, commonly used in weight loss formulations, so its use as an anti-irritant is not fully understood.

Another plant used for the same reason is *senduduk* (*Melastoma malabathricum, below*). Taken for womb healing and for the treatment of leucorrhea (excessive, foul discharge of the vagina), it grows wild virtually everywhere in Malaysia. The aqueous extract of the leaves contains analgesic, anti-inflammatory and anti-pyretic properties, so it is helpful in the relief of pain and inflammation as well.

The future is sure to see better formulations of such herbs, manufactured and packaged under strict guidelines, entering markets worldwide. Women's healthcare is improving as women assert themselves globally; with increased spending power and a desire for self-help and self-healing, such natural products are bound to gain ground.

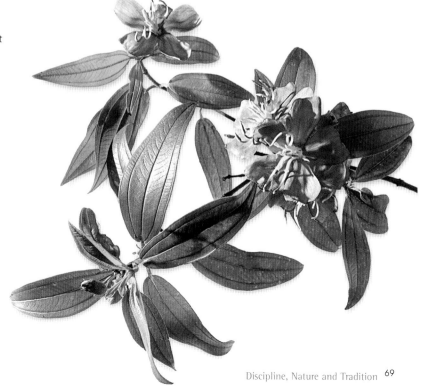

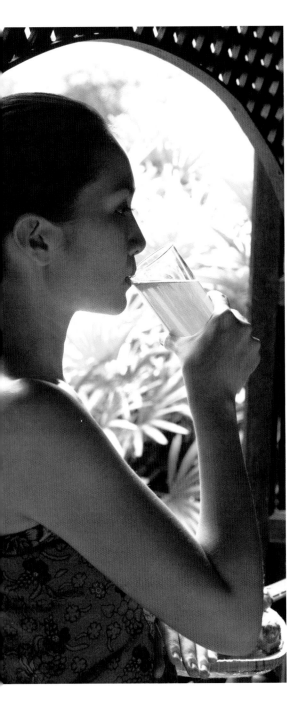

Herbal Remedies
for Nursing Mothers

Once a woman is out of confinement, she may be fully recovered physically from her birth and pregnancy, but she still faces many challenges. There may be difficulties with the baby and problems with the mother that still need to be dealt with, and, of course, Malay herbalism has an answer for most (if not all) such occurrences.

Mother's blues or *meroyan* is a case in point. While Western medicine often resorts to chemical help for post-natal depression, the Malays feel answers are to be found in the natural world. They believe that meroyan can have long-lasting effects in a woman's life cycle, so it needs to be attended to straight away.

Meroyan is thought to be caused by excessive wind entering the body. If this happens, the new mother is prone to bloating, chills, aches and depression—a condition known as *banyak angin*. If untreated, this irritability can lead to the mother experiencing erratic mood swings and depression in later life. To prevent this, she is prescribed with an antioxidant, anti-inflammatory herbal drink containing such plants as ginger, lemongrass, jerangau and other herbs. This concoction helps eliminate toxins, cleanses the blood, balances hormones and, hopefully, will be a life changer in the long term.

Young, and older, mothers often have problems producing enough milk for the baby's needs. So, of course, the Malays have formulated a wonderful milk and honey drink to help with this. Containing an extract of *selasih hitam* (*Ocimum tenuifloram*) and fenugreek, this drink is recommended with an intake of shark's meat to strengthen the mother's blood and its antibodies. In addition, some mothers are given boiled green beans, *turi*

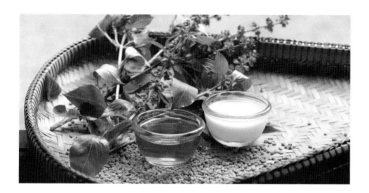

Meroyan is thought to be caused by excessive wind entering the body. If this happens, the new mother is prone to bloating, chills, aches and depression.

leaves (*Sesbania grandiflora*) and also soymilk to promote an abundant milk flow.

Naturally, there are also treatments for mothers who produce too much milk or have blocked milk flow or mastitis, as well as topical applications of roots and leaves to prevent cracked nipples and all the possible ailments that can plague breast-feeding mothers. There are also certain practices that couples are encouraged to undertake in the fields of family planning and infertility. Similarly, when couples want more children, there are certain folkloric traditions that are believed to be able to help them conceive either a girl or a boy!

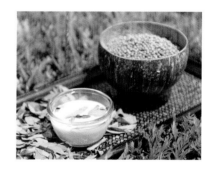

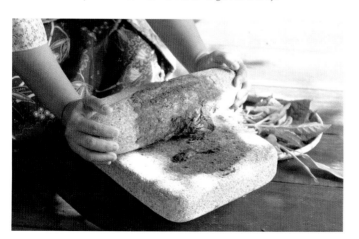

Opposite New mothers take an anti-inflammatory herbal drink, containing such plants as ginger, lemongrass, *jerangau* and other herbs.

Top Ingredients for a special milk and honey drink to help mothers produce more breast milk.

Above Green beans, *turi* leaves and soymilk promote milk flow.

Left Traditionally, herbal plants are ground to a paste to prepare a 'cooling' remedy for mastitis.

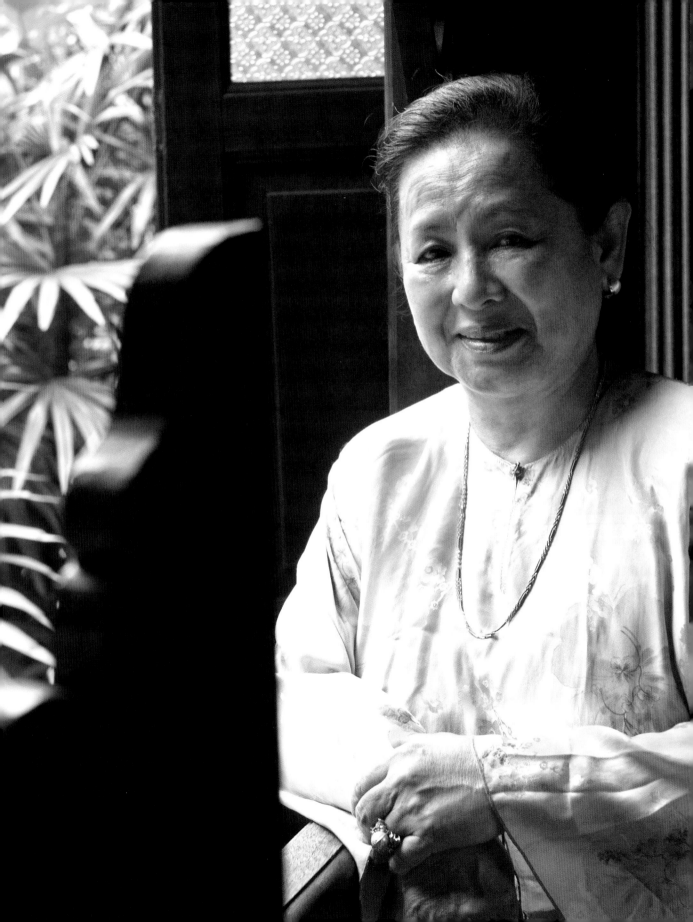

Mature Women:
Health Problems and Remedies

Hormonal imbalances are part and parcel of many women's lives, with some sailing through life without any problems and others finding themselves struck down with any number of complaints: tender or lumpy breasts, fibroids, endometriosis, premenstrual syndrome, infertility, difficulty in carrying a pregnancy to term, sudden weight gain, fatigue, irritability and depression, foggy thinking, water retention, memory loss, headache, migraine. . . the list is seemingly endless.

Most of these symptoms are caused by hormonal imbalances of one type or another, and, according to the Malay pharmacopeia, can be remedied. An excess of estrogen and deficiency of progesterone, leading to premenopausal syndrome is one problem that most women experience at some time in their lives. The Malays look at premenopausal syndrome as *penyakit melanuih*, a chronic ailment that is the result of a life lived out of balance. As such, there are a few golden rules that women are encouraged to follow: drink an hour before a meal and an hour after a meal, but not during meals or immediately after meals. This helps with bloating and liver complaints. To prevent chills and pain in muscles and joints, women are encouraged to avoid drinking iced water or bathing in icy cold water. Rather, they substitute, especially during menstruation, a refreshing ginger drink that includes pandan leaf, fenugreek, black seed and lemongrass, all sweetened with palm sugar. Betel leaf juice and tamarind juice once or twice during menstruation help with heavy flow and strengthen bones and muscles.

Combined with dry saunas and luluts, such practices are believed to strengthen and balance hormones and enhance

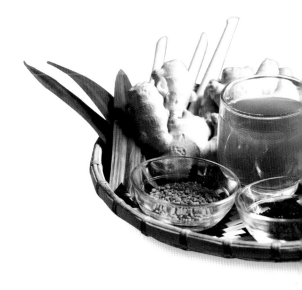

The Malays look at premenopausal syndrome as *penyakit melanuih*, a chronic ailment that is the result of a life lived out of balance.

Opposite Malay women tend to go through menopause with ease and grace.

Above Ginger drink taken during menstruation.

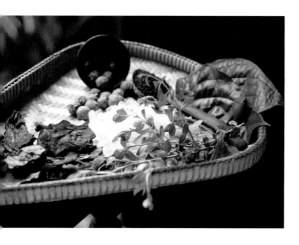

healthy reproductive organs. Women are also encouraged to practice a type of Malay exercise known as *senaman asak badan*. With poetic-sounding movement names—tiger movement, bird movement and snake movement, for example—such postures and repetitions help with muscle firmness and overall wellbeing.

In the Western world, a menopausal woman is frequently portrayed as someone who is irrational, depressed, unstable, unattractive and suffering from an abnormal medical complaint. In Malay society, however, women have accepted menopause as a necessary transition in life. They tend to go through this period with ease and grace and there is little mention of menopausal maladies afflicting women in Malay annals. Closer examination reveals that this is not the result of any special or magical concoction; rather, it's a combination of a life lived with discipline, traditional knowledge and natural products long before menopausal age is reached.

However, there are certain exercises, practices and remedies that women who are aged 50 and above are recommended to follow. Pelvic floor muscles need to be tightened regularly to prevent bladder and uterus prolapse; sitz baths and special washes for the intimate area are encouraged; sitting on a hot stone wrapped with *morinda* (or noni) leaves, betel leaves, fenugreek, ginger and black seed is recommended for those with back aches or a low uterus; and, held to be useful in cases of osteoporosis, is the practice of eating a traditional Malay dish of rice with *lemuni* (*Vitex negundo*), ginger, turmeric and *pegaga* (*Centella asiatica*). It's believed to abate the weakening and deterioration of the bones, common in menopausal women.

During menopause, many women complain that their skin takes a rapid turn for the worse. The force of gravity beckons,

Above Ingredients used for the anti-aging sitz bath.

Below Rice mixed with *lemuni*, ginger, turmeric and *pegaga*—a popular traditional Malay dish menopausal women are encouraged to eat.

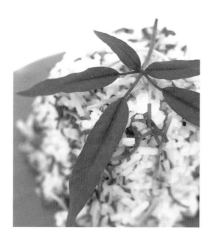

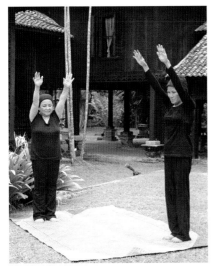
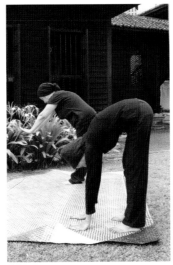
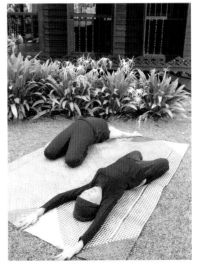
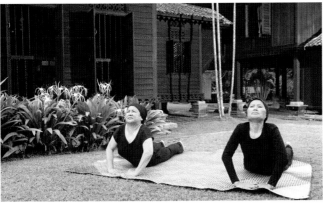
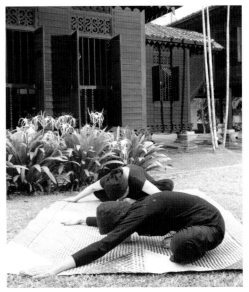
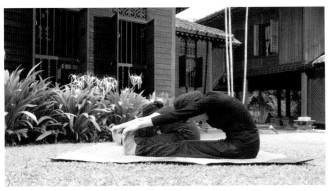

Clockwise from top left *Senaman asak badan* begins with arm stretches; other steps include the *harimau* (tiger) movement; *kuntum* (flower) movement; *burung* (bird) movement; *kucing* (cat) movement; and the *ular* (snake) movement.

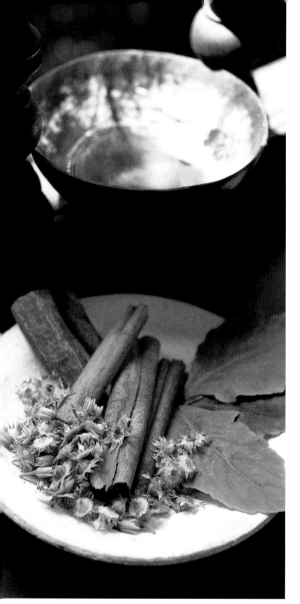

wrinkles become deeper, and the texture and condition of skin deteriorates. This is because the sebaceous glands gradually stop secreting sebum (oil) and the level of protein in the form of skin collagen decreases. A special herbal bath formulated specifically to help with skin pigmentation, age spots and blemishes is recommended; it also helps with excess body hair, another sign of menopause. Women make a scrub with *sintok* (*Cinnamomum sintoc*) and Kaffir lime and use it in the bath; this is followed with a herbal oil of cinnamon, *Mimusops elengi*, *nilam* (*Pogestemon cablin*) and coconut oil.

As estrogen levels drop, so does hair on the head. Menopausal women's hair often becomes thinner, in some cases chunks of hair fall out, and women often experience loss of self-esteem as a result. A wash of ripe morinda (or noni) fruit, Kaffir lime and sintok could be the answer; it seeps deep down into the roots of hair and strengthens follicles.

A Life of Balanced Self-care

It can be seen, therefore, that the Malay woman has many resources at her disposal. Expertise culled from generations of her forebears, all having gone through the same stages she experiences, is a great teacher. As all the remedies are natural, she doesn't have to worry about troublesome side effects; and, as most of the plants, herbs and roots she uses are close to hand, she doesn't have concerns about sourcing and obtaining them. Certainly, making the decoctions can be time-consuming, and results are definitively not seen overnight. But, a disciplined approach with constant vigilance and practice, leads to a healthy life well lived—a life in balance, where inner wellness is reflected in the outer appearance.

Above Herbal oil made of cinnamon and *Mimusops elengi*.

Opposite, above Patchouli plant.

Opposite, below Frangipani are often used in herbal and floral baths.

Scents and Sensibility

Malay women have long produced herbal cosmetics, steams, elixirs and powders with beautiful scents. The power of scent is well known, with certain fragrances making people productive and active and others calming or soothing the psyche. It is known that the olfactory nerve goes directly into the brain, so the sense of smell is both primary and extremely evocative. Scent triggers the release of neuro-chemicals in the body; these send messages to our brains to alter the way we feel.

Of course, the ancients have known this since time immemorial. When certain branches or twigs were thrown on to the fire, the aroma emitted from the smoke made people feel drowsy and peaceful. Hence, the word 'perfume'—derived from the Latin 'through smoke'—came into being. Similarly, holy or magic smoke (incense) has been used in most major religious rituals for centuries. Indian and Chinese cultures have a long history of meditation and incense burning and it's known that the Orang Asli in the Malay Peninsula have burned aromatic woods to appease the spirit world for millennia.

Aromatically scented materials such as agarwood (see page 35), frankincense and myrrh play important roles in religious ceremonies, rituals and in human courtship. Similarly, essential oils from many plants are

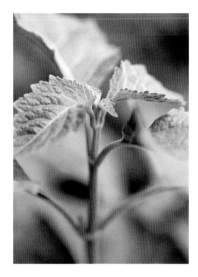

used today in the preparation of the fragrant components of scents, cosmetics, body creams and lotions, hair care treatments and air fresheners.

Take patchouli (*Pogostemon cablin*), for example. Known in Malay as *nilam*, dried patchouli leaves were traditionally used as a moth repellant in the textile industry. Patchouli, however, is better known for its essential oil that is both distinctive and extremely long lasting. This has made it a key ingredient in the formulation of fine perfumes and cosmetics. It's also commonly used in aromatherapy and massage oils for its relaxant attributes.

Frangipani (*Plumeria* sp.) is another favorite scent. Its local name is *kemboja*, coming from Cambodia or Kambuja, suggesting the flower's ancient links and origins. Its pretty white or pink blooms, with their strong, heady scent, are often used in herbal and floral baths in combination with other aromatics. Its leaves, when mashed into a paste, were used on boils, as was its milky white sap.

Citronella grass (*Cymbopogon nardus*), known as *serai wangi* in Malay, is another example of a strong-scented plant. Its essential oil, citronella oil—obtained through steam distillation of the stems and leaves of the plant—contains limonene, methyl isoeugenol, geraniol, citronellol and citronellal. The latter three are extensively used in soaps, perfumery, cosmetics and as a flavoring. In Malaysia, citronella oil is traditionally used as a component of herbal material in aromatherapy to revitalize new mothers during their confinement periods and as a mosquito repellant.

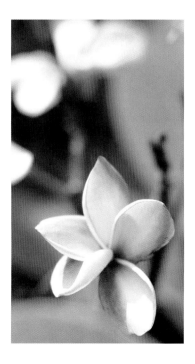

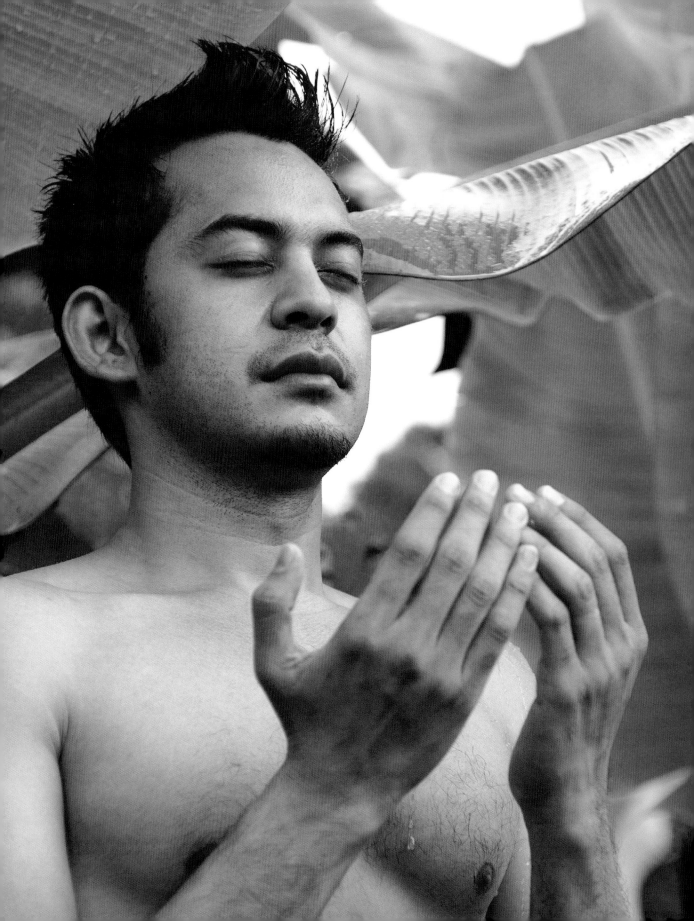

Vigor and Vitality
Men's Health in the Malay Tradition

In Malay tradition, it is not only women who are expected to look after their health and wellbeing throughout life. Men must concern themselves with their physical and emotional conditions as well. This is especially true after marriage, as, in the Malay world, matrimony is seen as a turning point in the life of a man. From this time on, he is expected to shoulder the responsibility not only for his own life, but for that of his wife, and eventually his children, too.

While some of the rituals a man needs to master are geared towards general strength and wellness, many are designed to enhance sexual prowess. Traditionally, Malay men were expected to father many children, so virility was especially desired. It was thought that a virile man was a healthy one: good health was equated with the size of a man's family.

Traditional Malay Exercise

Malays from all walks of life (farmers, fishermen, warriors and princes) have long practiced a series of bodily movements known as *senaman asak badan* to maintain, nourish, revitalize and prolong their lives. Combining breathing techniques with postures and movements, there are similarities between senaman asak badan and Indian yoga and Chinese tai chi.

Opposite Many of the rituals a Malay man needs to master are geared towards general strength and wellness, as well as enhancing virility.

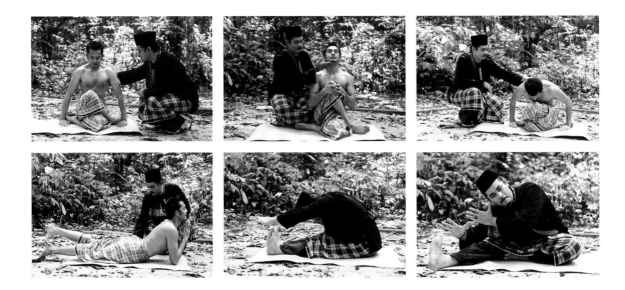

Usually performed at dawn or in the early morning, and sometimes combined with prayer, the exercises are therapeutic in nature. There are certain key postures (some of which are not unlike yoga *asanas*) and particular sequences, many of which are named after animals or movements they resemble. These names are often taken from the natural world, for example, *senaman ular* (snake posture) and *senaman harimau* (tiger posture). These postures have different styles, but are unified in a common aim of improving flexibility, agility, endurance and strength.

Sessions often begin with some gentle warm-up exercises with inhalations and exhalations of breath to bring a better sense of clarity and focus and to enhance endurance. This is followed by individual postures or a moving sequence of such postures, with emphasis placed on specific breathing patterns. The general aim is to promote a relaxed and supple body and a peaceful state of mind. Additionally, these exercises are thought to enhance sexuality and masculinity. Sessions usually end with some floor exercises that help the body to cool down.

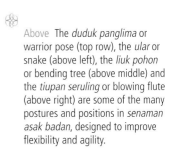

Above The *duduk panglima* or warrior pose (top row), the *ular* or snake (above left), the *liuk pohon* or bending tree (above middle) and the *tiupan seruling* or blowing flute (above right) are some of the many postures and positions in *senaman asak badan*, designed to improve flexibility and agility.

Traditional Herbals for Male Vitality

In the Malay world, the status of a man's health is measured by how virile he is. It is a common belief in Asia that male sexual prowess and stamina is closely related to a man's spirit, so men are keen to feed this spirit in order to improve libido, endurance and strength.

Two particular herbs, *ubi jaga* (*below*) and *tongkat ali* (*right and far right*), have traditionally been consumed to increase overall energy, enhance sexual potency, strengthen erections, boost the metabolism and improve fertility. Originally taken in powdered form or as a tonic or decoction of root chips, they are increasingly consumed in the form of premixed coffee or tea sachets and as pills, capsules or liquid formulations.

Ubi jaga's botanical name is *Smilax myosotiflora* DC and it was customarily chewed with betel leaf and areca nut as an aphrodisiac. It is believed to increase blood circulation and was also taken for syphilis.

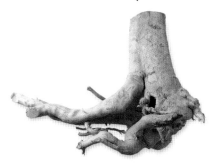

When used in combination with tongkat ali (*Eurycoma longifolia*), it was regarded as a potent force. Unfortunately, there is little hard scientific evidence as to how exactly it works.

Tongkat ali, on the other hand, has undergone several trials. With oral administration of tongkat ali extract to rats, it has been noted that the rats showed an increase in testosterone level and a growth of the seminal vesicle and ventral prostate. Studies also showed increased sexual arousal. Even though it tastes bitter, tongkat ali is a firm favorite among Malay males, who swear by its efficacy.

Certainly, market demand for such botanicals is high and there is no reason why they should not be consumed in more user-friendly forms, as long as they comply with safety and quality requirements and are registered with drug regulatory agencies.

The rich biodiversity of tropical Malaysian flora offers a huge opportunity for the manufacturing of products from such plants with high bio-medically active compounds. Traditional people living close to the ancient rainforest habitats of these tropical plants have harnessed their properties for centuries. Their efficacy is now being validated by scientists and doctors in the modern era.

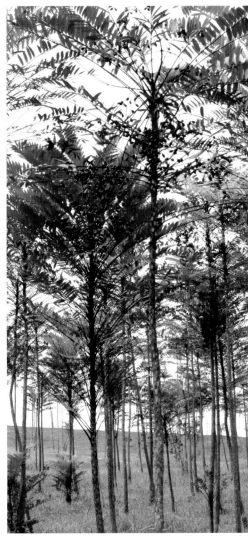

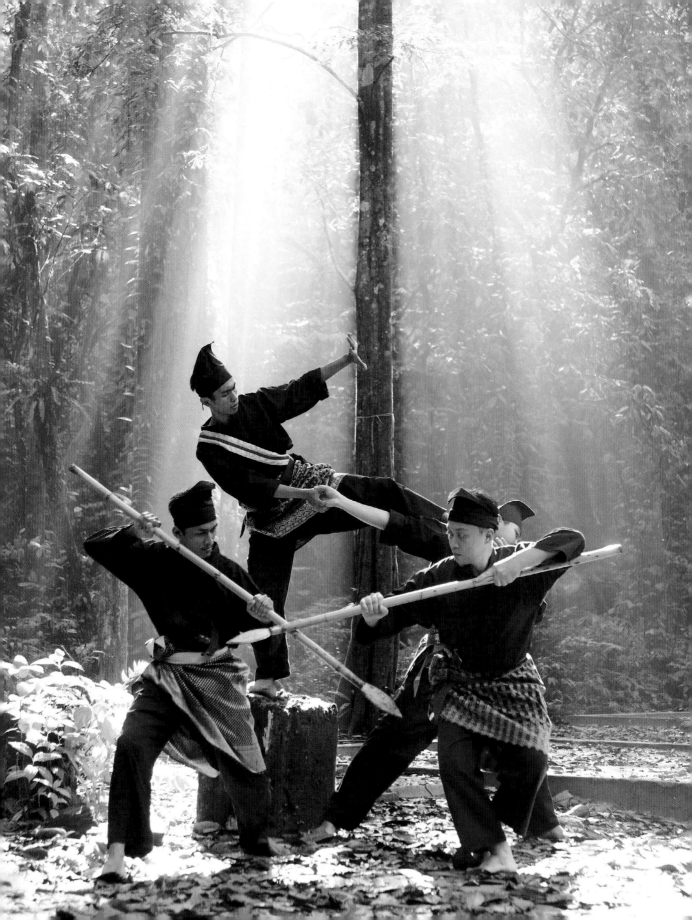

Silat, the Malay Martial Art

Another form of exercise is called silat. Although not as well known globally as some of the Chinese and Japanese martial arts, silat is widely practiced in Malaysia. A synthesis of powerful martial art movements and graceful ritual dance, there are over 400 silat forms in the Southeast Asian region, with about 200 regularly practiced in Peninsular Malaysia. Silat Gayong, Silat Lincah and Silat Cekak are the three main schools, with the first being the most popular.

Silat is an extremely elegant and restrained style of martial art. Putting a premium on self-control and discipline before violence, it compels the participant to develop a body of ritualized skills that harness potential feelings of aggression. Combining breath, movement and energy techniques, with self-awareness and empowerment, it expresses some of the more important principles of *adat*, the unwritten codes of conduct in traditional Malay society. In adat, the ideal is a life of self-control, discipline and honor; this can be obtained through silat, where an ordinary mortal can transform himself into a famed warrior.

Malay silat forms contain two basic ritual components: the system of *pantang larang* or personal taboos designed to prepare a person physically and mentally for a course in self-defense, and the principles of combining psycho-physical acts (*zahir batin*) towards achieving final perfection. Comprising a series of *kunci* or 'locks' and *pukul* or 'strikes' with both hands and feet, movements can be both vigorous and dynamic as well as gentle and slow. Most work towards immobilizing an opponent rather than causing pain—and all combine to improve the practitioner's health and foster fulfillment on more than the physical level.

Silat, an extremely elegant and restrained style of martial art, combines breath, movement and energy techniques.

Opposite Silat compels the participant to develop a body of ritualized skills that harness potential feelings of aggression.

Below An extremely elegant and restrained martial art, silat places an emphasis on self-control and discipline.

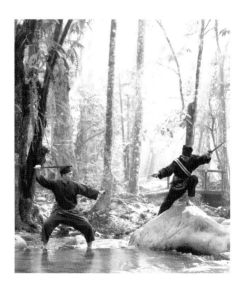

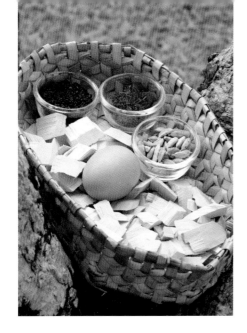

Herbal Cleansing

As well as exercising body and mind, men are traditionally encouraged to undergo powerful detoxification as well. The Malay custom of drinking a concoction of boiled roots and rhizomes including betel (*Piper betle*), *temu lawak* (*Curcuma xanthorrhiza* Roxb.), ginger, *misai kucing* (*Orthosiphon stamineus*), *ketapang* (*Terminalia catappa*) and red ginger (*Zingiber officinale* Var. *rubrum*) was believed to enhance virility and sexual desire. The mixture has antioxidant properties, and, when stirred with pure honey, is fairly palatable. It is still taken all over Malaysia today.

The same can be said of *majun kuat*, a bitter decoction of *koma-koma* or saffron, black seed, cardamom, testosterone-enhancing *tongkat ali* (*Eurycoma longifolia*) and chicken egg. Taken as a purgative, it is believed to improve digestion, enhance immune function and promote cell development. Reducing fat and stimulating white blood cell production, it encourages muscle build-up, virility and the development of strong and healthy sperm.

In fact, there are many such drinks in the Malay almanac. All tend to focus on boosting the libido, strengthening the nervous system and promoting healthy bodily systems such as blood and lymph circulation. As is usual, they focus on both internal functions and external appearance.

Another discipline is the *mandi wap* or herbal steam bath, a ritual that a man is expected to practice once a week. Its primary function is to break up fats and mucus that may have accumulated in the body. Made with boiled banana leaves, fenugreek, black seed, coriander and tongkat ali, it is believed to improve the circulation of the blood and lead to increased vigor and vitality.

Above *Majun kuat* comprises saffron, black seed, cardamom, testosterone-enhancing *tongkat ali* and chicken egg.

Below *Mandi wap*, or herbal steam bath, consisting of *tongkat ali* and black seed, should be practiced once a week to break up accumulated fats in the body.

Blockbuster Drugs: Natural Not Synthetic

Many allopathic drugs in use today trace their roots back to plants. Over the years, manufactured synthetic substitutes of the original compounds have replaced the natural substances. However, there are a number of plant species whose natural compounds continue to be used to this day. Similarly, some are still being researched by some of the big pharmaceutical companies.

Internationally, examples would include such life-saving and significant plants as the anti-malarial Chinese wormwood (*Artemisia annua*) from southern China; the cinchona (*Cinchona officinalis*), originally from the Peruvian Amazon; the anti-cancer rosy periwinkle (*Catharanthus roseus*) from Madagascar; and another valuable anti-carcinogen, taxol, initially extracted from the bark of yew trees from America's Pacific Northwest and now, more sustainably, from the leaves of a range of yew species.

Blockbusters from the Malaysian rainforest include the anti-cancer *bintangor* from Peninsular Malaysia and Sarawak, and the testosterone-enhancing *tongkat ali*, also indigenous to Malaysia.

Bintangor or *Calophyllum* spp. (*right*) is a genus of the family Guttiferae, to which the popular mangosteen also belongs. In May 1987, Harvard University carried out a joint collection with the Forest Department in Sarawak in order to search for new plants with tumor-arresting properties. A national cancer institute funded the study to find new drugs to combat cancer and AIDS. Plant specimen collections were made in a lowland mixed dipterocarp forest near Bintulu, an alluvial forest near the Gunung Mulu National Park, the limestone hills near Bau, and a peat swamp and *kerangas* forest near Lundu. Emphasis during collection was placed on flowering plants, species from as wide a variety of families and genera as possible, and plants reputed to have medicinal uses locally. The breakthrough came in late 1991, when the extracts from at least two species of bintangor exhibited positive activity against HIV.

Tongkat ali or *Eurycoma longifolia*, also known as longjack, is a flowering plant in the family Simaroubaceae, native to Malaysia and parts of

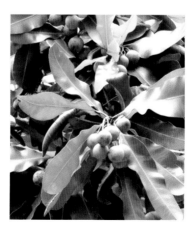

neighboring Indonesia. It is a small evergreen tree, growing to around 15 meters in height, with spirally arranged pinnate leaves. The flowers are dioecious, with male and female flowers on different trees. The fruit is green, ripening to dark red, about 1 to 2 centimeters in length and 0.5 to 1 centimeter across.

This species is popular locally for its alleged testosterone-enhancing ability and, as a result, has been included in some herbal supplements for bodybuilders. Historically, Malaysians have utilized the herb for its suggested anti-malarial, anti-pyretic, anti-ulcer, cytotoxic and aphrodisiac properties.

Some scientific studies suggest that tongkat ali enhances sexual characteristics and performance in animals. In other studies, tongkat ali extract has been shown to induce cell death or aptosis in breast-cancer cells and to be toxic to lung-cancer cells. A 2003 study showed that *Eurycoma longifolia* resulted in increased muscle strength and size when compared to a placebo. This may demonstrate the anabolic properties of tongkat ali, but more research is needed.

While further scientific research is still being carried out on this species, the pure extract of the active compound has now been introduced to the international market. It is also blended with a number of beverages that are sold to enhance both sexual and athletic prowess.

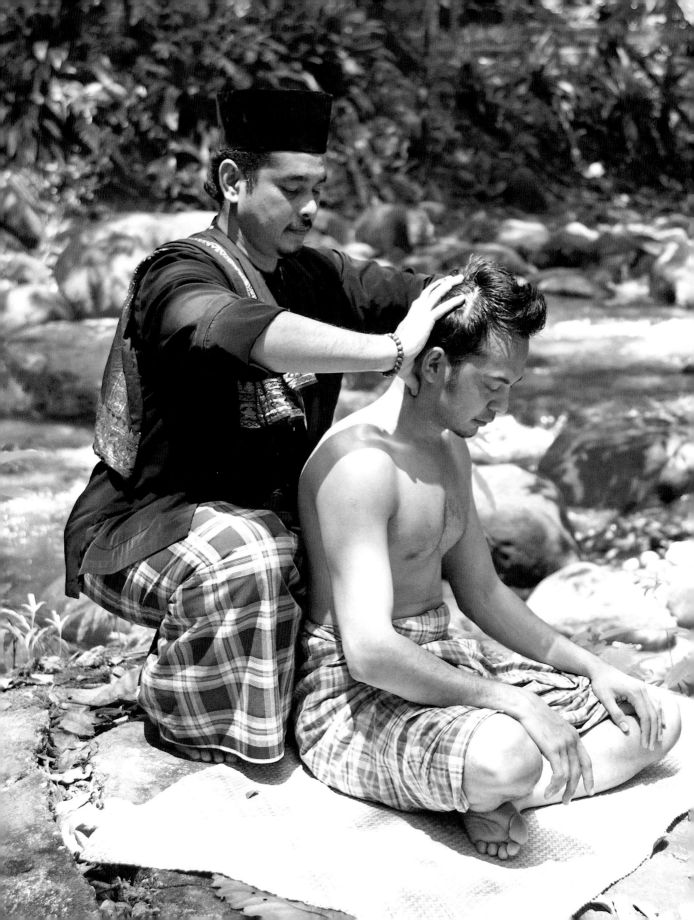

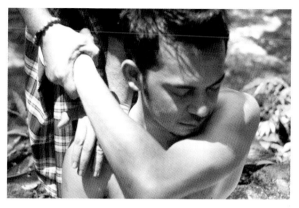
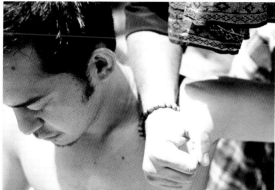

Traditional Massage

Another helpful step in improving energy and libido levels is through the traditional Malay massage known as *urutan tenaga batin*. Using a specially brewed herbal oil of cloves, cardamom, galangal, fenugreek, lemongrass, gingers and *jerangau* (*Acorus calamus*), it is performed only on the back, pelvic area and inner thighs. Particular strokes, designed to increase blood circulation and energy flows, are used. The massage needs to be performed by an expert, as one wrong movement can cause harm.

Another type of massage that men usually perform on themselves in conjunction with their exercise sessions is *urutan asak*. Generally practiced at dawn in order to harness the energy of the early morning, it is combined with the slightly unsavory sounding oil known as *minyak lintah* or leech oil. Made from leeches brewed in coconut oil, tongkat ali and the aphrodisiac creeper *ubi jaga* (*Smilax myosotiflora*), it is believed to stimulate the nervous system. The oil is smeared over the whole body, particularly in the lower back area, the gluteal muscles in the buttocks, the knees and the genital area, then the man massages his body with upward strokes. These are designed to facilitate smooth blood flow and soften tense nerves, all the while stimulating the body's reserves.

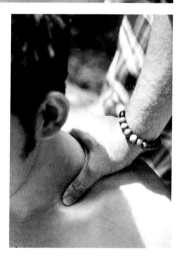

Opposite The traditional Malay massage *urutan tenaga batin* improves energy and libido levels. It must be performed by a trained expert.

Above Stretching and massage techniques used for common shoulder and neck problems such as strains, sprains, aches, pains and poor posture.

A Research Partnership on Malaysian Herbs

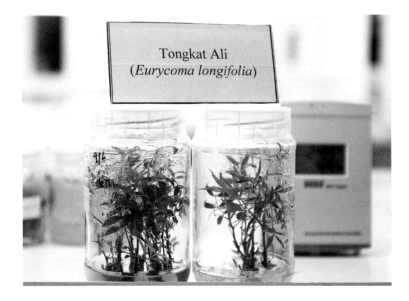

As part of a wide collaboration between Malaysia and the Massachusetts Institute of Technology (MIT), research was conducted on selected Malaysian herbs at MIT and a number of leading research centers throughout Malaysia.

As the medicinal ingredients in *tongkat ali* (*Eurycoma longifolia*)—Malaysia's wonder plant for male vitality and general energy—are found most potently in its root, the plant is destroyed whenever a medicinal harvest is done. With seven or so years being the youngest age at which tongkat ali can be harvested, there is clearly a need for sustainable harvesting methods to be developed. So, the Malaysia–MIT research program focused on increasing production of tongkat ali by lab methods: *in vivo* and *in vitro* cultivation procedures.

This high-level scientific exchange resulted in the chemical fingerprinting of tongkat ali being accomplished— a process by which all of its chemical ingredients, their proportions and interactions are known. This is very useful as a standard for producing future stocks for cultivation that have similar medicinal properties to wild stocks. From this, a standardization protocol was established, enabling the production of consistently high-quality tongkat ali products.

And there were new discoveries. Two new bioactive components from extracts of tongkat ali were isolated and characterized. One of these is now used as a reference standard for the standardization of all tongkat ali products.

The MIT and Malaysian scientists found that laboratory propagation of tongkat ali was indeed possible. Now whole plants have been generated using cellular material from tongkat ali. And a method has been developed to cultivate just the root in a lab setting, so that large scale production of the active chemicals may be extracted without endangering wild stocks of this important plant.

DNA studies have evaluated the genetic diversity of tongkat ali in its natural habitat, and a number of variants that are highly receptive to cultivation and regeneration have been identified, thus allowing for diversification and enhancement of the tongkat ali gene pool.

From this fruitful international partnership, two patents have been filed for tongkat ali, relating to its bioactive fractions and to its genetic markers.

Tongkat Ali
(*Eurycoma longifolia*)

A Healthy Diet

Of course, in keeping with the Malay ideas about cooling winds, men are advised to avoid certain foods that are believed to be particularly 'cooling'. These include 'cold' foods and drinks such as young coconut water, sugar cane juice, soursop juice, iced water, vegetables that are creepers, venomous fish, bamboo shoots, goat's liver, cold rice and duck eggs.

On the other hand, most other vegetables are encouraged, as are dates, olives, garlic, ginger, honey, milk, beef, rice, eggs and salt. Honey, known as the 'enemy of diseases' in Malay lore, is considered an especially powerful anti-aging tool, especially useful for those who have passed middle age. It is thought to be a natural energizer, and men are encouraged to take it whenever possible. Straight from the honeycomb is best, but commercial honey is also considered efficacious. One particular formula is thought to enhance physical strength: a mix of honey, egg and saffron. Recommended for newly weds and for those with a low libido, it's considered a guaranteed pick-me-up.

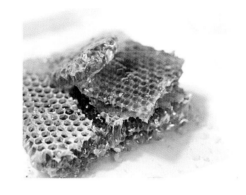

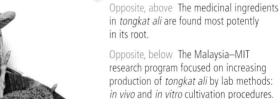

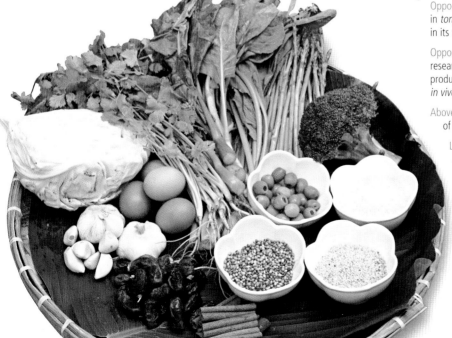

Opposite, above The medicinal ingredients in *tongkat ali* are found most potently in its root.

Opposite, below The Malaysia–MIT research program focused on increasing production of *tongkat ali* by lab methods: *in vivo* and *in vitro* cultivation procedures.

Above Honey is known as the 'enemy of disease'.

Left Some of the foods men are encouraged to eat include eggs, garlic and dates.

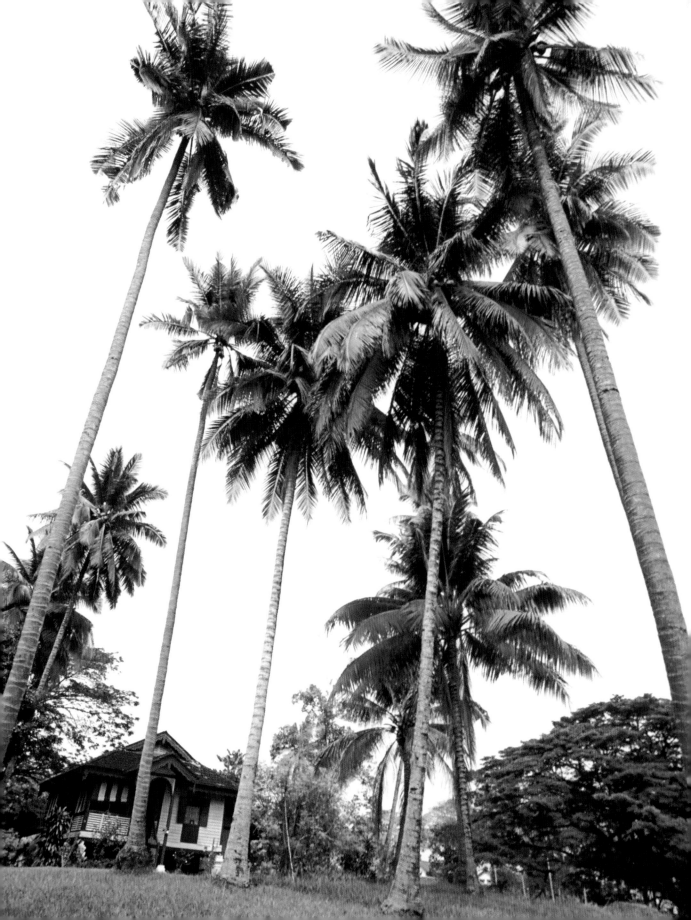

From Rainforest to Kitchen
Health Traditions in the Malay Family

The idea that we are what we eat, or rather we are what our ancestors ate, is not a new one. Science has proved the direct link between a wholesome diet and a healthy body and mind; today, nobody would argue that a packet of crisps is better for you than a fresh green salad. But what's interesting is that many traditional societies have known about the benefits of a healthy diet—and a healthy environment—for centuries. They certainly didn't analyze it, agonize over it or question it. In all probability, they simply lived it.

Malaysia is a case in point. Traditional *kampung* (village) life was truly anchored in the surrounding environment. Living in harmony with the natural world, in sync with the dramatic cycles of monsoon and subsequent sunshine, drawing on the rich variety of tropical plants and trees all around, was never questioned. It simply was. It is only since the advent of today's sedentary lifestyle, with consumption of fast food and chemical beverages and the attendant woes of stress, tension and illness, that people have begun to see (and understand) the benefits of this ancient way of life.

Historically, people in the Malay Peninsula viewed human life as a series of cycles and phases. From the time a child is in the womb, through to birth, inclusion in the family and growth through to old age, he or she followed a set pattern. With each

Opposite Traditional *kampung* (village) life draws on the natural environment.

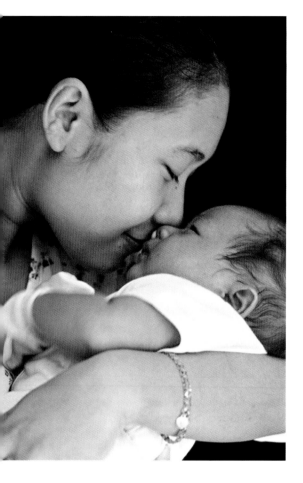

stage came change; with each cycle of life, there were different needs. All these needs were catered for through nature.

And, of course, by the mother in the family! Mothers took responsibility for the health and emotional needs of aged relatives, spouses, children and grandchildren. They provided everything that was needed in the domestic sphere. As such, they were known as *ibu*, a term that translates both as 'source' and 'mother'. Appropriately enough, the tropical rainforest plants prepared by mothers to maintain health and manage illness in their families, are themselves accorded the status of ibu.

Thus, the common Malay saying, *syurga di telapak kaki ibu* ('heaven is at the mother's feet'), reflects the deepest respect for a woman, and for a mother in particular. The mother is seen as the source of power, of healing energy, the lifeblood of the family and the environment in which she resides.

A Rich Repository of Health-Giving Ingredients

In the past, food, clothing, income, medicine, shelter and sustenance, health and welfare were all provided for by Malaysia's vast natural reserves—its rainforests. Among the oldest on earth, these forests originated 70 million years ago in the Pleistocene Era and have a biological richness and diversity unequalled even by those of the Amazon or Africa. Naturally, they're home to hundreds—if not thousands—of medicinal plants. Within an arm's reach of most rural kampung homes, such plants are also found growing in household gardens too.

Almost a century ago, the renowned British botanist, Isaac Henry Burkill, observed that medicinal gardens were common

Above The common Malay saying, *syurga di telapak kaki ibu* ('heaven is at the mother's feet'), reflects the deep respect for a mother in the Malay culture.

Opposite The mangosteen fruit is prized for its taste and antioxidant properties.

in Malay villages. Indeed, the knowledge of plants for health and healing among Malay kampung dwellers provided rich source material for Burkill's epic work, *A Dictionary of the Economic Products of the Malay Peninsula*. What Burkill discovered was that these gardens were not only living pharmacies, but handy sources of nutrition and beauty enhancement too.

Take the exotic mangosteen (*Garcinia mangostana*). Native to the Malay Peninsula, this fruit is somewhere between the size of a golf ball and a tennis ball and resembles a white mandarin inside when its pulpy purple shell has been peeled away. Mangosteens are hugely popular in Asia for their rare flavor, somewhere between a passion fruit and a peach. Ancient seafaring traders took mangosteens to Sri Lanka, where they have thrived and become prized for their delicious, delicate taste as well as for their value in medicine and beauty preparations. They've also spread to other Asian countries too.

The tree is highly versatile: Malay women make a preparation from mangosteen peel to enhance the complexion. The tannin in mangosteen shells is also extracted as a dye for textiles, while the coming-of-age tradition for Malay boys sees the use of an infusion of mangosteen leaves combined with unripe banana and a little balsam. More recently, the exotic mangosteen has been found to contain potent antioxidants known as xanthones; these give immune systems a boost and also combat viral and bacterial infections. The mangosteen is clearly a valuable fruit tree to have growing in the family garden.

Medicinal gardens in Malay villages were not only living pharmacies, but handy sources of nutrition and beauty enhancement.

The Ginger Family: Malaysia's Herbal Superstars

There are more than 1,400 species of plants listed in the Zingiberaceae family, but only a few are used for culinary and traditional therapeutic purposes in Malaysia. However, of these few, they are used time and again in a variety of combinations, with common ginger and turmeric (see page 108) probably being the most popular. The large number of chemical constituents present in ginger and turmeric illustrates the opportunities that further scientific research into the gingers offers. For example, the discovery of active compounds can be utilized to treat various ailments such as cancer and HIV.

Contrary to popular misconceptions, ginger rhizomes have myriad different shapes, colors, flavors and properties. Usually dug up and ground into a fine paste or powder, or mixed and boiled with other ingredients for their cumulative effect, they are the undisputed superstars of the Malay healing world.

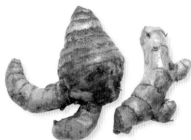

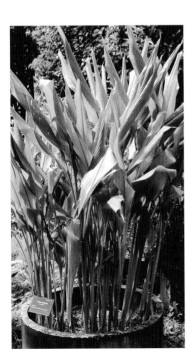

:: ***Temu lawak*** (*Curcuma xanthorrhiza* Roxb., *above and left*) is a popular ingredient among Malaysians of Indonesian origin as it is widely used in Java in traditional tonics. Believed to have anti-aging properties, it is used in literally hundreds of healing prescriptions: as a postpartum infusion or concoction to hasten contraction of the uterus; mixed with tamarind juice for relief from rheumatism; for kidney problems, asthma, gastric problems, constipation and headache. It is also indicated for treatment of cancer especially during the early stages or after surgery, and is popular in facial and body care applications. Malaysian housewives have been using temu lawak for centuries. And, in the 19th century, the rhizome's success in liver and gallstone treatments led to large quantities being exported to Holland where they were made into infusions and drunk daily.

:: Common **ginger** (*below*), known locally as *halia* and scientifically as *Zingiber officinale*, is found in nearly every kitchen in Malaysia. Used for flavoring, it is a common ingredient in soups prescribed for fevers, colds and nausea. Due to its anti-spasmodic properties, ginger is widely used to treat rheumatism, colic and flatulence. It's a common practice to apply a lotion prepared from ginger, vinegar and coconut oil on the abdomen post partum to help restore the stomach muscles to their pre-pregnancy state. It's also a popular ingredient in teas; grated ginger, honey and quail's egg is a general tonic and aphrodisiac, while a decoction of ginger is used to treat stomach ache, nausea and vomiting associated with motion sickness, pregnancy and cancer chemotherapy. Massage oil with ginger extracts is also widely used.

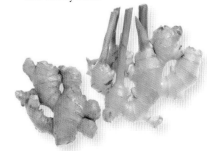

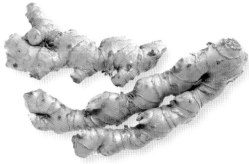

Extracts of ginger show the presence of more than 400 chemical constituents, too lengthy to list. Suffice it to say that gingerols are the magic ingredient!

:: *Lempuyang wangi* or *Zingiber aromaticum* (*above and right*) is a fragrant ginger popular in tonics prepared principally for warming the body and increasing muscle flexibility. It is also used for treating sore throat and whooping cough, and, when mixed with Java pepper (*Piper retrofractum*), is used as a treatment for edema. Expressed juice of the rhizomes mixed with salt is taken for treating hemorrhoids, while a treatment for anemia is a decoction of the rhizomes with palm sugar.

Despite its many therapeutic uses, fragrant ginger came to the spotlight in 1999 when a formulation of the extracts of fragrant ginger, temu lawak, *temu ireng* (*Curcuma aeruginosa*), bael fruit (*Aegle marmelos*), honey and sugar, was mixed with chicken feed to promote resistance to bird flu. The extract of the fragrant ginger has also been found to have anti-cancer, anti-inflammatory and anti-HIV activities. Its anti-cancer activity is attributed to its suppression of free radical generation.

:: **Galangal** or *lengkuas* (*Alpinia galanga* or *Languas galanga, below*) is widely used in Southeast Asian cooking to marinate beef, chicken or mutton for the traditional satay dish. It possesses carminative and stomachic properties, so is used to treat nausea, flatulence, dyspepsia, catarrh and enteritis. Sometimes, it is enough to consume meals cooked with galangal to alleviate the problems. A decoction of galangal in the bath water is believed to help with rheumatism, and, due to its tonic and anti-bacterial properties, it is

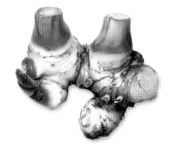

used in veterinary and homeopathic medicines. Recently, it was reported that galangal extract was found to kill cancer cells and promote healthy cells adept at protecting themselves from carcinogens.

:: Galangal's close relative, *Kaempferia galanga* or lesser galangal (*cekur* or *kencur*), has a strong flavor and aroma, so when it is used in cooking, it is only used sparingly. Traditionally, it is one of the ingredients in the postpartum *bengkung* wrap, while in traditional Chinese medicine, a decoction or powder of galangal is used to treat indigestion, cold, pectoral and abdominal pains, headache and toothache. It is also valued for its skin protectant properties.

The discovery of novel chemical constituents in the Zingiberaceae family (curcumin, zerumbone, gingerols and other constituents that have yet to be determined) is creating a great deal of interest in the scientific community. New studies and more research are already taking place, thereby promoting some of Malaysia's herbal traditions. Similarly, recent findings indicating galangal as an anti-cancer rhizome may help to promote the health-giving aspects of many Asian cuisines. People in the region have been eating the gingers for centuries—for flavor, aroma and their health-giving properties—and they haven't been doing so for nothing.

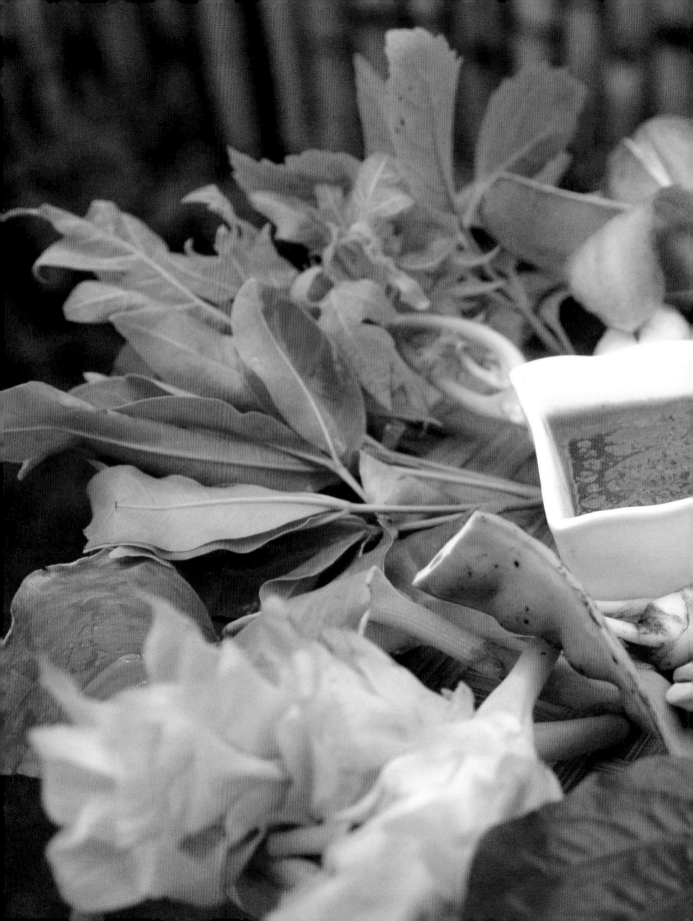

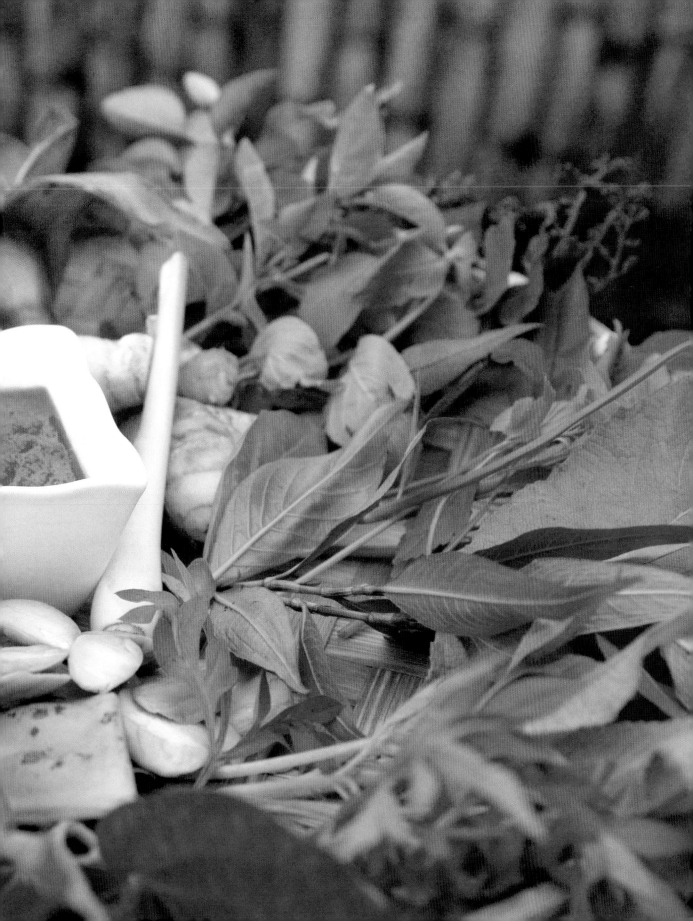

Ulam

Where Food Meets Medicine

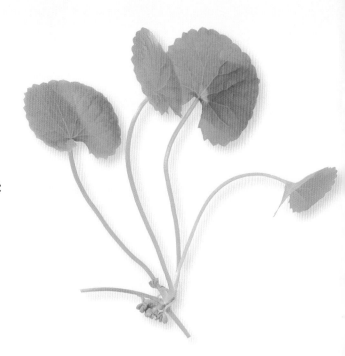

A preparation that combines food, medicine and beauty
is the widely popular Malay herbal salad known as *ulam*.
Traditionally, villagers collected the young shoots or *pucuk*
of a variety of locally growing plants to make the freshest,
most delicate ulam.

Today, bustling night markets, wet markets and
even supermarkets sell these herbal salad ingredients to
city dwellers who cherish the traditions of their village
forebears. In rural areas, ulam plants are still gathered from
the wild or grown within the village vicinity, much as they
have been for centuries.

To understand the medicinal knowledge of
the *kampungs*, let us consider a small tree native to
Southeast Asia known poetically in Malay
as *daun tenggek burung*, literally 'the
leaf where the bird rests'.

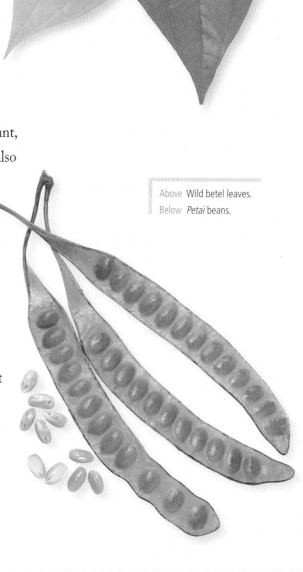

Botanically, this is *Euodia ridleyi* and it's used by mothers in rural Malaysia for managing stomach problems. When life is lived close to nature, gastric infections are common, and, in children, often serious. This bitter plant is included in ulam, both for its taste and its efficacy.

Also added to ulam is wild betel leaf or *Piper sarmentosum*, a member of the pepper family. Known as *kaduk* in Malay, it grows near fences and watercourses throughout the tropics. It's useful in the treatment of coughs and colds, and as it is an expectorant, it clears the chest of excess mucus. The whole plant is also used to treat fever.

It's not just leaves that go into ulam. Malaysia's bright green *petai* bean (*Parkia speciosa*), although an acquired taste, is a popular ulam ingredient. Sold in bunches of full bean pods and in bags of shelled beans, it contains three natural sugars—sucrose, fructose and glucose. Petai also contains tryptophan, a protein that is converted by the body into serotonin; so not only will a petai ulam boost energy, it will produce a smile as well. And if a mellow mood were not enough to induce better health, petai is also high in potassium and low in salt.

Above Wild betel leaves.
Below *Petai* beans.

The list goes on . . . ! A small, mustard-smelling plant known to the Malays as *pokok ketumpangan air* ('shining bush') and to the world of botany as *Peperomia pellucida* is a familiar companion in ulam. It grows naturally in wet areas—abundant in the tropics—and is used in Malay medicine for fever, headache, backache and general weakness.

As well as adding a mustard flavor to the already spicy herbal salad, this little gem has anti-inflammatory, anti-bacterial and analgesic properties. It's often accompanied by *temu lawak*, a type of turmeric that has a large pink flower and yellow root. Although glorious in a tropical garden, its utility is prized more than its beauty: it has an aromatic fragrance that hints at its camphor oil component and is a traditional remedy for stiff muscles and jaundice.

Above *Pokok ketumpangan air.*

Right *Temu lawak* roots.

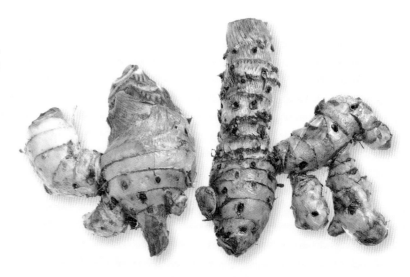

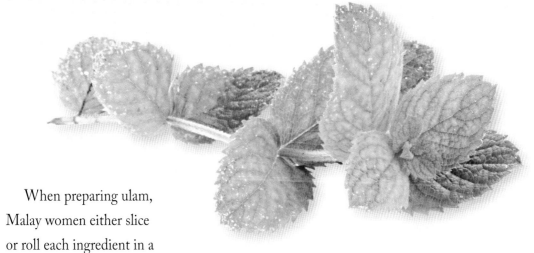

When preparing ulam, Malay women either slice or roll each ingredient in a way that best brings out its flavor. *Daun pudina* (mint leaves) are chopped finely to release their zesty aroma and taste, while *laksa* leaves are rolled, then sliced very finely. The handsome torch ginger with its crowned flame-like flower (*Etlingera elatior*) is sliced in rings to add a light piquancy to the leafy ingredients, while *pegaga* (*Centella asiatica*) is rolled into a ball with the stem serving as a tie. It is then chewed much like a plug of tobacco, so as to extract every drop of its goodness.

Other common aromatic ulam herbs include local varieties of mint, *tulsi* or holy basil, lemongrass, turmeric leaves and Kaffir lime leaves. These are combined with vegetables such as long green beans and cucumber. In keeping with the cultural principle of not eating too much of the same thing during one particular period of time, mothers vary ulam ingredients regularly. What doesn't change, though, are the foods that accompany ulam: a fermented shrimp and chili sauce known as *sambal belacan*, salted fish, dried prawns, fish crackers and fried grated coconut.

Top Mint leaves.
Below Torch ginger.

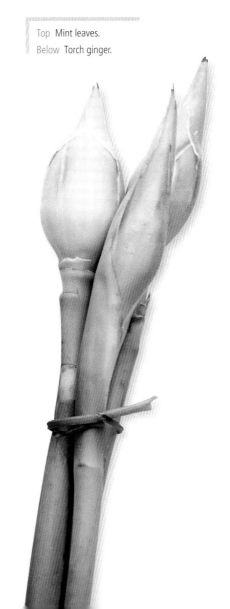

Ulam and its Antioxidant Activities

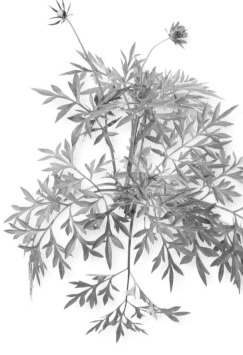

Antioxidants are in the news a lot these days—but what are they and why are they important?

An antioxidant is a molecule that can slow or prevent the oxidation of other molecules. Rust is a process of oxidation—and we know what it can do to a car. The same process occurs with oxygen particles known as free radicals; they form branching chain reactions and lead to damage in the human body. They've been linked with cardiovascular disease, various forms of cancer, inflammatory conditions including rheumatism and many other medical concerns. Naturally, good antioxidants are important as a means of preventing this type of damage.

In a recent study of traditional vegetables used in *ulam*, the following were shown to have significant antioxidant activity; they also have other uses too.

:: *Belimbing* or carambola (*Averrhoa carambola*) is a member of the star-fruit family. As is often the case, this pretty fruit has multiple uses. The most acidic species are used to clean the blade of the *kris* (Malay dagger), while medicinally it's used in an infusion for coughs and as a tonic after childbirth.

:: *Gelang pasir* or common purslane (*Portulaca oleracea*), in addition to being a popular ingredient in ulam, is also used as a de-worming agent.

:: *Terung meranti* or black nightshade (*Solanum nigrum*), taken in small amounts, can be a good laxative and a sedative, though its fruit in high doses is toxic. New research shows it can remove toxic polychlorinated biphenyls (PCBs) from contaminated soil, making it a potentially good prospect for farming in degraded areas.

:: *Daun kesum* or Vietnamese coriander (*below*), also known as *laksa* leaf (*Persicaria tenella*), is listed in the Global Compendium of Weeds. However, its popularity as a Malay ulam and an essential ingredient in laksa noodles throughout Southeast Asia just goes to show how relative the concept of 'weed' is.

:: *Ulam raja* or 'king's salad' (*Cosmos caudatus, above*) was brought by the Spanish from tropical America, via the Philippines, to Southeast Asia. As they sailed across the Pacific, the Spanish used it as a vegetable to sustain themselves during the long journey. Ulam raja has been found to have anti-fungal and anti-bacterial effects. Malaysians also believe it has anti-aging properties or *awet muda*, and that it tones up blood circulation, strengthens the bones, and promotes fresh breath.

:: *Temu pauh* or 'mango ginger' (*Curcuma mangga*) is a member of the ginger family Zingiberaceae and is closely related to turmeric. It is yet another potent antioxidant in the ulam mix.

:: *Selasih* or sweet basil (*Ocimum basilicum*) is linked with antioxidant activity. Research has shown that sweet basil has valuable anti-aging, anti-cancer, anti-viral and anti-microbial properties.

:: *Daun gajus* or cashew leaves (*Anacardium occidentale*) are eaten raw in ulam when young as the mature leaves are toxic. They have an anti-diabetic effect as they lower blood sugar levels.

Health Across Ages and Stages

Life in the tropics is always dramatic, with extremely hot dry months alternating with steamy downpours and high humidity. Societies have adapted their lives to this natural cycle— planting, tending and harvesting crops at certain times of the year and using seasonal produce as and when it becomes available. They've also adapted their family cycles to the cycles of nature, benefiting from her extravagant abundance for general wellbeing, healthcare and beauty. And, because ritual is a part of life in Malaysia, each stage of life is celebrated with certain rites of passage. Many times, these have health and wellbeing connotations as well.

Birth and Early Years

The birth of a child in Asia is always greeted with great excitement. Children are a confirmation of the continuity of the family lineage and provide a source of joy, companionship and security for their parents' old age.

The first stage of life is accompanied by a complex array of traditions and practices designed to enhance the baby's start in life. Building the immune system, calming the infant, and creating balance and happiness through touch and nourishment are key. Management of the pregnant mother, the baby and the post-natal mother is given over to a highly respected member of the community— the midwife or *bidan*. The bidan holds an influential position among women in Malay society. Recognized as a *dukun* or healer, she often acts as a bridal attendant or matron of honor at weddings and serves as an intermediary in betrothal ceremonies.

Because ritual is a part of life in Malaysia, each stage of life is celebrated with certain rites of passage. Many times, these have health and wellbeing connotations.

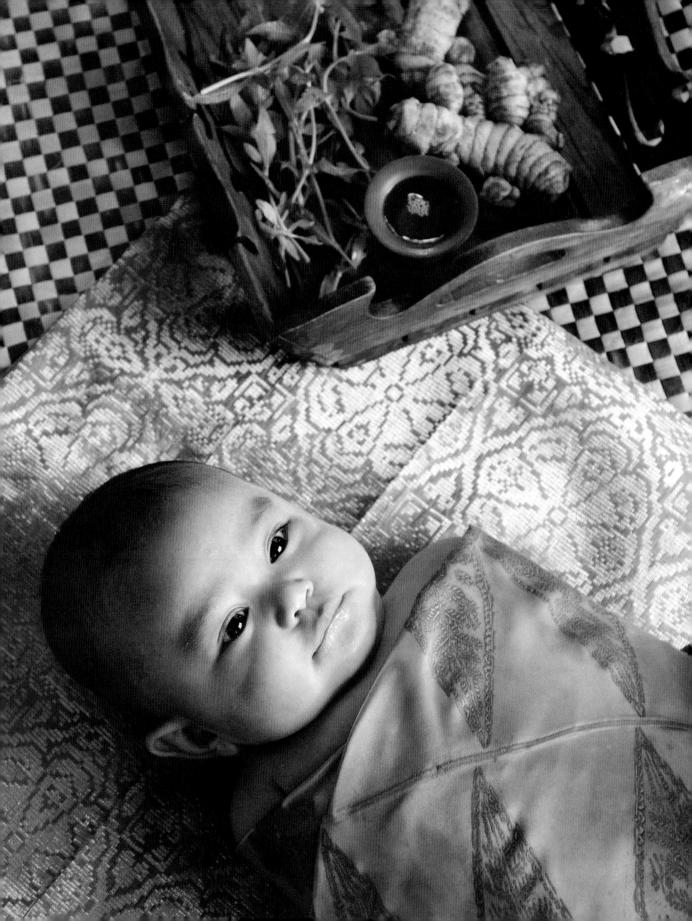

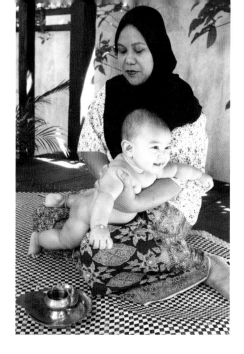

The bidan's body of knowledge—in herbalism, therapeutic practices such as massage, and culinary matters—is often orally passed down through the generations. As is the case with other healers, bidan often beget bidan, thereby preventing centuries of wisdom from being lost.

Therapeutic massage plays an important role in all stages of life, but particularly in the care of mother and baby. Prior to birth, the midwife uses a range of herbal oils to massage the mother, while babies are massaged daily to strengthen muscles, improve blood circulation and give the immune system a boost. An aromatic, vitalizing oil made from coconut oil, nutmeg oil, turmeric, ginger, shallots and black pepper is used.

Massage oil is rubbed onto a baby's scalp to help with cradle cap and is used on the abdomen, back and legs to prevent and relieve colic. Grated and dried turmeric mixed with coconut oil on the fontanel is said to protect the baby from colds. Baby girls are covered from head to toe with a form of natural body powder to care for their skin. Made from starch flour, ground rice, dried turmeric, dried galangal, pandan leaves and jasmine flowers, it is mixed with water and splashed onto every part of the body. It's a wonderful, scented example of a traditional and enduring early beauty skin care treatment.

Either 30 or 100 days after the birth, a special ceremony known as *cukur jambul* is held. During this, the newborn baby's head is shaved in a purification rite, then gently massaged with an emollient, antiseptic oil of turmeric and *keremak* leaves (*Alternanthera sessilis* L.). Mixed with linseed oil, this soothes the scalp and promotes healthy hair growth. A more local tradition is to use the mother's milk mixed with finely powdered star gooseberry (*Sauropus albicans*) and *minyak sapi* or ghee—it's considered a surefire recipe for thick glossy hair.

Opposite The *cukur jambul* ceremony is held either 30 or 100 days after the birth of the baby.

Above Babies are massaged daily to strengthen muscles and improve blood circulation.

Below Baby massage oil made from coconut oil, nutmeg oil, turmeric, ginger, shallots and black pepper.

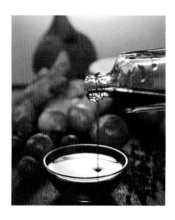

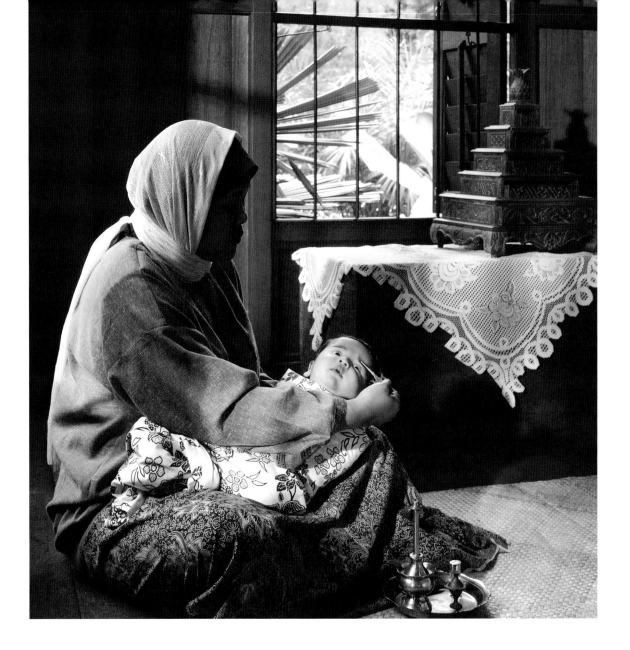

In another natural beauty treatment, the bidan shapes and darkens a baby's eyebrows by using an extract from the butterfly pea flower (*Clitoria ternatea*). Believed to promote healthy eyes and long curly eyelashes, mother's milk (high in immunological content) is commonly used for eye drops and as a gentle rub along the eyelash. Another popular eyelash beautifier that also prevents eye infections is homemade kohl eyeliner: made from ground almond, carbon, cuprum dioxide,

Above The *bidan* shapes and darkens a baby's eyebrows.

Opposite, above A warm betel leaf compress is administered on a baby boy.

Opposite, below The baby's daily bath water is infused with betel leaves, pandan leaves and willow leaves.

ochre, ash, malachite and chrysocolla, it's a common sight around the eyes of small Malay children.

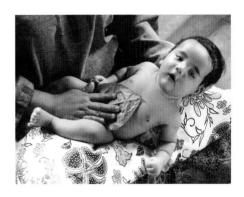

As boys are believed to be more prone to umbilical hernias than girls, they are often treated with a warmed betel leaf compress on the stomach, pelvic area, back and genitals. Three to seven betel leaves are gently heated on a hot river stone or charcoal embers. The leaves are then placed on the body after it has been rubbed with coconut oil infused with nutmeg, lemongrass and coriander seeds. Soothing and warming for the baby, as well as effective in preventing flatulence and hernias, the leaves are usually applied twice a day.

All this touching, rubbing, massaging, carrying and hugging provides warmth, support and love, as well as therapeutic care to infants. The daily bath is another highly tactile activity that also has symbolic significance. Much more than quick dip and a splash, it's given in water that has been boiled and infused with betel leaves, pandan leaves, willow leaves (*Salix babylonica*), *keranda* fruit (*Carissa carandas* L.), black seed (*Nigella sativa*) and turmeric. This bath is believed to prevent jaundice, convulsions and skin allergies. Additionally, the baby is held firmly by the bidan and gently hoisted up and down seven times. Call it an early form of exercise, or a muscle strengthening activity, it's a delight for tiny tots.

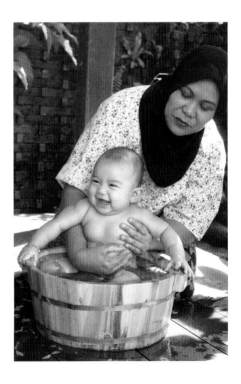

Similarly delightful is the application of a special homemade baby powder that protects sensitive skin. Prepared from ground *bedak sejuk* (pearl rice) that has been soaked in water for weeks or months, sago flour blended with turmeric powder or a white clay powder, it is soft, antiseptic and non-irritating. Afterwards the baby, wrapped up firmly in a soft cotton cloth, feels clean, comforted and cared for.

Turmeric: A Mother's Choice

Connecting the link between mother (*ibu*) as the source of nurturing and the rainforest as a source of life, some plants in Malay medicine have had the word ibu incorporated into their names.

Turmeric (*Curcuma longa* or *kunyit* in Malay), a highly prized ingredient in post-natal, skin and digestive health, is one such example. Appropriately enough, turmeric's main rhizome is more often referred to as ibu kunyit.

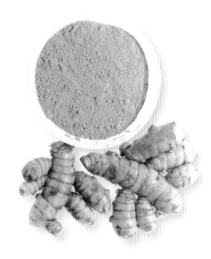

Echoing the Malay mother's faith in the range of ibu kunyit's healing properties, turmeric is also used in many Ayurvedic, traditional Chinese medicinal and allopathic remedies. The US National Institutes of Health currently has four clinical trials in progress studying the effects of curcumin, the active ingredient in turmeric. It is believed that it may have real benefits in the treatment of pancreatic and colorectal cancer, multiple myeloma and even Alzheimer's disease.

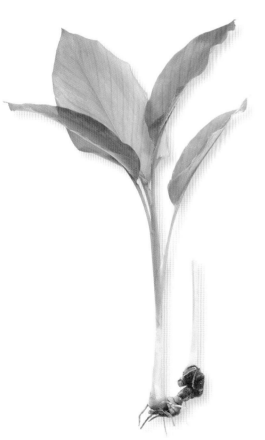

In traditional Malay home healing, the rhizome is the main part used, although the leaves are sometimes used to flavor and enhance the aroma in cooking. The flowers are normally eaten raw as *ulam* and are believed to cleanse the blood. The young rhizomes are also eaten raw as a postpartum protective treatment. Mixed with lime, the rhizome is topically applied to treat bruises, sprains, wounds and leech bites, while a decoction is taken for treating diarrhea, dysentery, flatulence, dyspepsia, colic, jaundice and amenorrhea. It is also drunk to kill worms in the stomach and has found its way into beauty care as a dilapatory.

Science has now shown that turmeric contains up to 5 percent essential oil and about 3 percent curcumin. The essential oil has been shown to have anti-inflammatory, anti-fungal and anti-bacterial properties, while petroleum ether extract of turmeric possesses anti-inflammatory and anti-fertility properties. Various scientific studies on curcumin, a polyphenol extracted from turmeric, have revealed anti-bacterial, anti-protozoan, anti-viral, anti-fibrotic, hypolipemic, hypochlesteremic, hypoglycemic, anti-coagulant, antioxidant, anti-tumor, and anti-carcinogenic properties. Ar-turmerone, another extract from the rhizomes, possesses anti-venom activity.

Curcumin is currently available in pure form and it is expected to be developed into a novel drug in the near future.

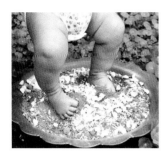

Opposite, above Turmeric powder and rhizomes.

Opposite, below Turmeric plant.

Above The *tijak bumi*, or 'earth step-ping', ceremony signifies the begin-ning of the baby boy's development of muscular and physical strength.

Although today's Malay families do seek out and follow the treatments prescribed by Western medicine, they often complement these modern treatments with their own age-old remedies.

There's one other childhood rite that needs to be mentioned: the *tijak bumi* or 'earth stepping' ceremony held just before a baby boy stands or formally goes outside the house. It signifies the beginning of the development of the muscular and physical strength that the little boy needs to hone for his steady progression into manhood and involves a ritual in which he takes his first tentative steps on a bronze, silver or golden tray filled with earth, yellow rice and *bertih* (toasted unhusked rice). Afterwards, he's bathed in cooling water enlivened with Kaffir lime and fed a little saffron or yellow glutinous rice, as a mark of thanksgiving. The tijak bumi is a joyous event and, depending on the resources of the family, can involve many guests.

As the child grows and matures, he or she gradually becomes aware of his or her own needs. Guided by both parents, girls and boys rise to the challenges of adolescence and maturity. However, many still continue to live in extended families and rely on the ibu's knowledge of general healthcare. Be it fever, chickenpox, cuts or more severe injuries, the Malay mother tends to her children by adding healing plants to meals and using them directly as medicine. Although today's Malay families do seek out and follow the treatments prescribed by Western medicine, they often complement these modern treatments with their own age-old remedies.

Common Ailments, Uncommon Remedies

In the tropics, fevers are common in childhood. Sometimes they're indicators of a serious tropical disease such as malaria or dengue, but often they are transient expressions of a viral or bacterial infection. In the West, oral medicine is often

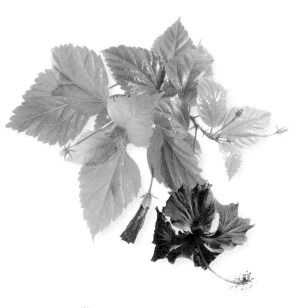

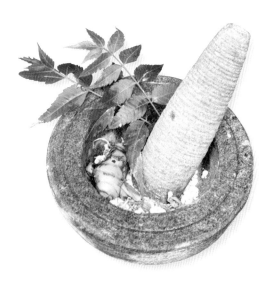

prescribed, but in the Malay tradition herbal decoctions or drinks and all-over medications are used to cool, soothe and heal. For non-threatening fevers, the home garden once again acts as a vitalizing source. Leaves from the hibiscus—whose glorious red blossom is Malaysia's national flower—are made into an extract to which is added pounded crepe ginger leaves (*Costus speciosus*) and cooling rice powder. Designed to have an overall cooling effect, the mixture is applied over the entire body.

In the case of chickenpox—during which itchy, angry pustules cover the body—the mother fries uncooked rice in a pan without oil until it is golden yellow, then soaks it in water. A handful of bedak sejuk (a specially prepared paste of soaked rice and pandan leaves) is added along with some pounded neem leaves (*Azadirachta indica*) and turmeric; when it becomes soft, this paste is applied to the spotty areas. Neem, a potent anti-viral, is also used as a fumigant to clear the air and drive out airborne forms of the virus from the family home.

Some other approaches to common family ailments include managing hemorrhoids and constipation by drinking twice daily a hot water extract, or decoction, of the stem from the betel leaf plant. Another drink for the same purpose is prepared from the calyx of *Hibiscus sabdariffa*, or roselle, known to the Malays as *asam susur*. *Daun kesum* (*Persicaria tenella*)—commonly found in swampy areas and also known as laksa leaves—is multi-faceted too. Used variously to relieve indigestion, bloating, dandruff and constipation, a drink of kesum is also given to pregnant women for general health and protection.

Because of the backbreaking nature of farm work in rural Malaysia, backache is a common complaint. For this, the pretty betel nut (*Areca catechu*) serves as a readily-available remedy.

Scented Resin

Among the many rich natural products of Malaysia, benzoin resin was long known to the ancient world as a kind of incense. The name benzoin is derived via Portuguese from the Arabic *luban jawi*, a translation of 'Java frankincense'. In antiquity, the term '*Jawi*' was generally used by Arab navigators to refer to the Malay Archipelago in general, so it's clear that early Arab traders knew where the resin came from. In fact, as early as 1350, the great Moroccan traveler Ibn Battuta recorded: 'After a voyage of 25 days we arrived at the islands of Sumatra, which give their name to the incense al-luban al-Jawi.' The term was taken up by the Portuguese in the 14th century, and from their version, *beijoim*, comes the modern benzoin.

In actuality, benzoin is the resin from any of several varieties of small trees in the family Styracaceae.

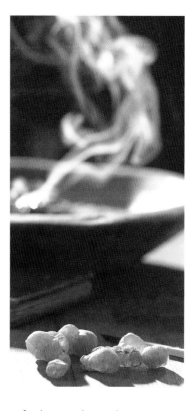

Indigenous to the highlands of Malaysia, it flourishes at around 1,500 meters above sea level, especially in primary rainforest. In addition to being a source of incense, it has long been recognized as a perfume and as a medicinal ingredient. Today two main varieties are cultivated: *Styrax benzoin* and the more common *Styrax paralleloneurum*.

Styrax, called *kemenyan* in Malay, has long been part of the traditional Islamic pharmacopeia. It is listed by the 11th century Persian scholar Ibn Sina, known in the West as Avicenna, as a dental restorative. It is similarly mentioned in the 17th century Dutch *Amsterdammer Apotheek*. Tincture of benzoin (benzoin resin dissolved in alcohol) and other derived versions, including the celebrated Friar's Balsam, were highly esteemed in 19th-century Europe as cosmetics, as well as for their anti-bacterial properties. Today tincture of benzoin is generally used in first aid for small injuries, as it acts as a disinfectant and local anesthetic and also promotes healing. It can be added to boiling water which, when inhaled, has a soothing effect on the lungs and bronchia, facilitating recovery from the common cold, bronchitis and asthma.

The antibiotic activity of benzoin resin seems mostly due to its abundant benzoic acid and benzoic acid esters, which are named after the resin; other less well-known secondary compounds such as lignans like pinoresinol are probably significant as well.

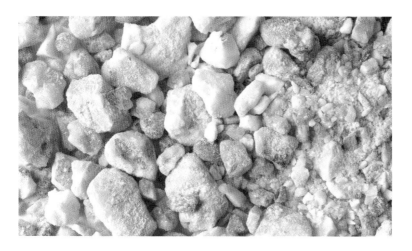

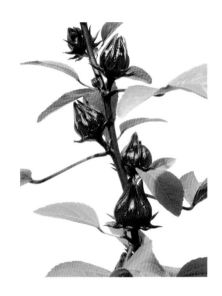

Above *Asam susur*, commonly known as roselle.

Below *Ikan haruan* is used to hasten the healing of wounds.

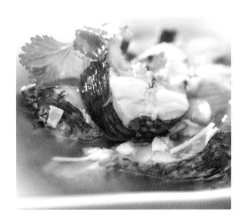

Known in Malay as *pinang* (its abundance gave rise to the name of the island of Penang), it is washed, ground to a pulp and mixed with coconut oil. The mixture is heated gently in a pan and then applied, with considerable reported relief, onto the back. As the heat and healing properties permeate deep down through the subcutaneous layers of the skin, they penetrate aching muscles and joints, all the while coaxing the pain away in waves.

Common cuts, wounds and burns are variously treated with a whole range of traditional concoctions, decoctions, pastes and poultices. Fascinatingly, Malaysia's snakehead fish—*ikan haruan, Channa striatus*—is used as a healing ingredient. Given in a soup to women after childbirth, ikan haruan has long been held to heal internal injuries resulting from delivery. Recent studies by Malaysian scientists have found high levels of the omega-3 fatty acid DHA (*docosahexaenoic acid*) in three species of this fish; this, they say, explains the centuries-old use of this fish in reducing pain and inflammation and promoting wound healing.

Whatever the complaint, there seems to be a cure. Or, if not a total cure, an alleviator of pain or a preventer of illness. Whether they are cultivated in the garden or gathered from the nearby rainforest, plants comprise part of an ancient and effective wellspring of healing knowledge. Naturally, they can double up as beauty ingredients or a tasty dinner for that matter. It's just one of the reasons many metropolitan Malaysians head home to their kampungs for special occasions. After all, there's nothing like ibu's home cooking: it keeps the doctor away, tastes delicious and is a reminder of that most precious of times, the days of long past country childhoods.

Culinary Herbs with Health Benefits

It is estimated that there are over 2,000 plant species with medicinal value in Malaysia. Naturally, not all are commonly used, but plenty find their way into prescriptions for health and beauty. A significant number are also used in cooking, as Malaysians often eat particular foods for their health benefits. The most common culinary herbs include peppermint, pandanus leaf, turmeric leaves (*Curcuma longa*), lemongrass (*Cymbopogon citratus*), Kaffir lime leaves (*Citrus hystrix*) and curry leaf (*Murraya koenigii*). In addition to imparting aroma and flavor to dishes, these herbs are also known to have therapeutic properties.

Pandanus or *pandan* (*Pandanus amaryllifolius*; *P. odoratus, below left*) is widely used in cooking and confectionaries in Malaysia. Both the leaf and juice are used as a flavoring agent and colorant, including to flavor drinking water. Pandan's characteristic aroma is caused by the same compound and flavor that gives white bread,

jasmine rice and basmati rice their typical smell. So, it is often used to impart a fragrance into rice, meat and fish dishes. In addition to tasting good, it is used to lower blood pressure, as a diuretic and to help ameliorate the symptoms of diabetes.

The young cluster of flowers arranged on the stem of torch ginger (*Etlingera elatior, right*) is another common culinary ingredient that finds its way into *laksa*, curries and mixed vegetable dishes. It gives that sour, aromatic, spicy and tangy taste characteristic of many Malay popular dishes and can also be consumed raw in *ulam* (see pages 96-102).

Unsurprisingly, it is also a versatile healing plant: a decoction of young shoots is taken as a postpartum treatment to reduce body odor, with the edible but sour mature fruits reputed to help with hypertension. Earaches are often treated with a decoction, while the young leaves are used to clean wounds. Scientists put

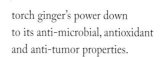

torch ginger's power down to its anti-microbial, antioxidant and anti-tumor properties.

Another common culinary plant in Malaysia, indeed all over Asia, is lemongrass or *serai* (*below right*). Used in fish, prawn and chicken dishes, it imparts a lemony taste and aroma to food. Traditionally, the leaves are used in an aromatic bath for women after childbirth. This is designed to reduce body odor and swelling and improve blood circulation. A lemongrass decoction is also used to treat boils, cuts and wounds, while an infusion of the leaves is helpful in treating digestive troubles, stress, toothache and swollen gums. Essential oil extracted from the stems and leaves finds many uses in aromatherapy and cosmetics. Therapeutically, the versatile lemongrass oil is analgesic, anti-depressant, anti-microbial, antipyretic, antiseptic, astringent, bactericidal, carminative, deodorant, diuretic, fungicidal and more. It is also used as a sedative and tonic.

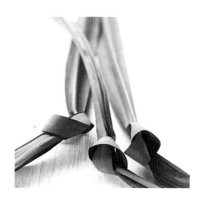

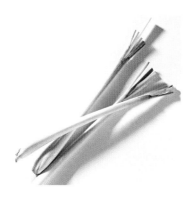

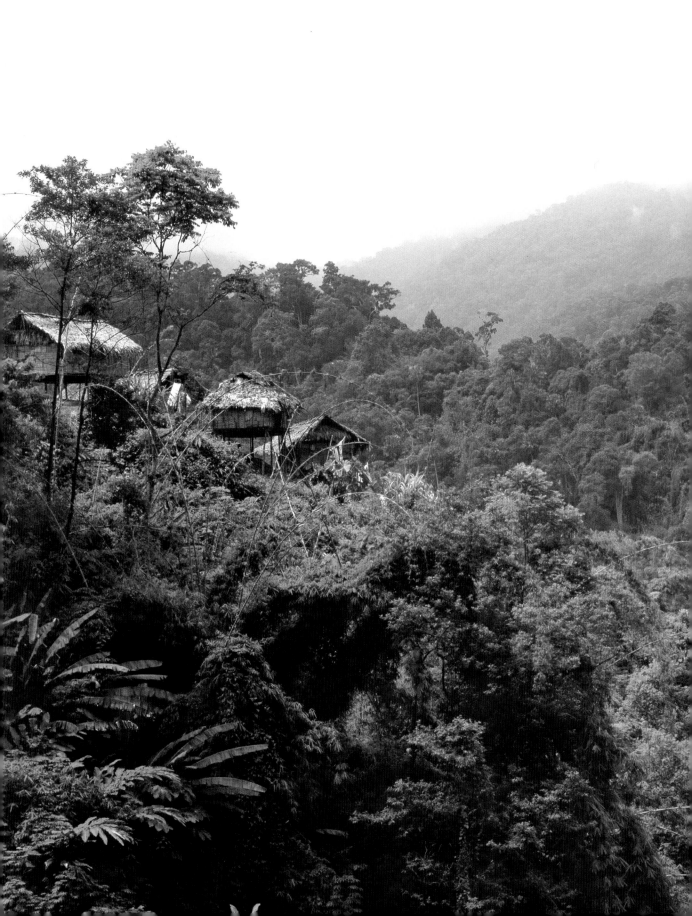

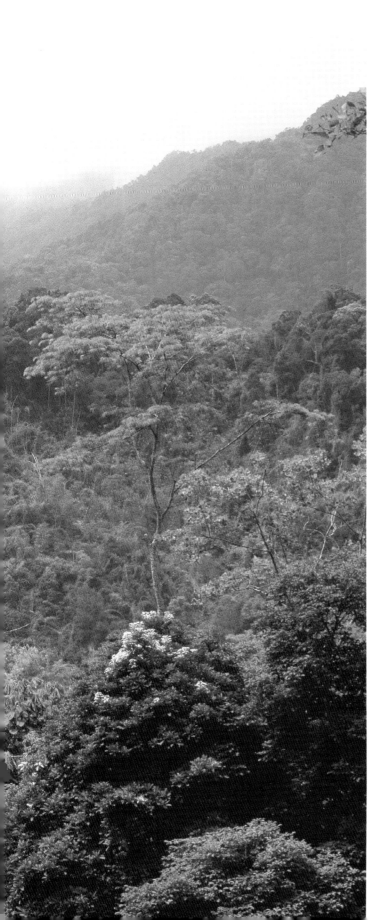

Healing Traditions and their Adaptations

Modern-day Malaysian society is a mix of races, cultures and religions. As such, its healing traditions have roots in a number of different sources: the healthcare practices of the Orang Asli or indigenous tribal peoples, the Malays, the Indo-Buddhist civilizations of South Asia, the Islamic civilization of Arabia and the civilizations of China and East Asia. Each and every one has left its mark on today's herbal healthcare practices. Malaysia presents itself to the world as 'truly Asia': this is reflected in its globalized healing approach and multifarious rituals and therapies.

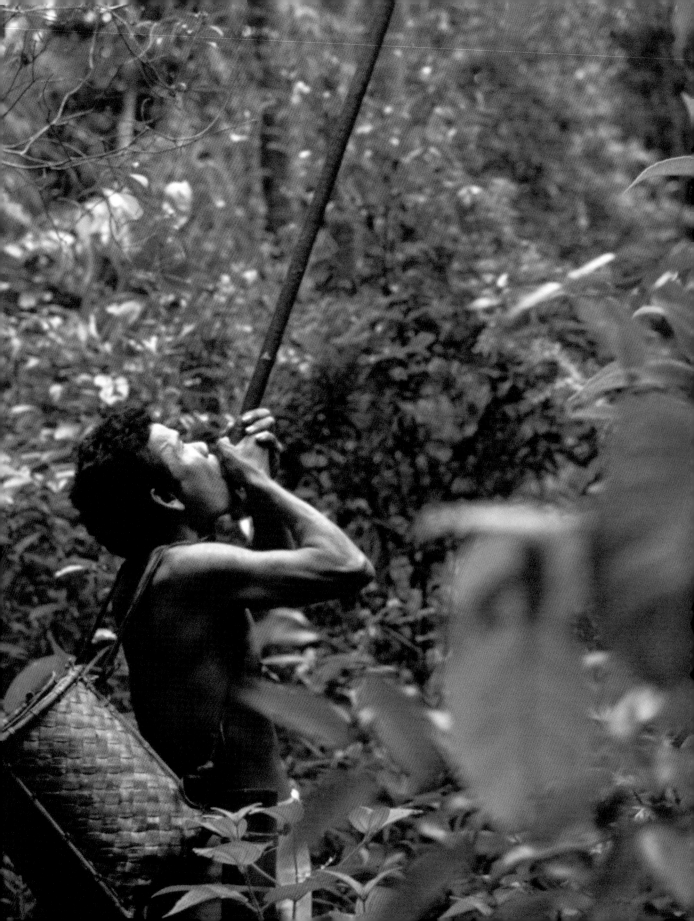

Ancient Peoples, Effective Healing
The Orang Asli

It is thought that the world's rainforests are home to around two-thirds of all of the animal and plant species on earth, and it has been estimated that many hundreds of millions of species of plants, insects and microorganisms still remain undiscovered.

They are also home, in Peninsular Malaysia, to the people who are known as the Orang Asli or 'original people', a term which refers to the country's indigenous peoples, the earliest of whom have a 60,000-year presence on the Malay Peninsula. Not typically homogenous today, the Orang Asli are broadly divided into three groups—Negritos, Senoi and Aboriginal Malay— which are further divided into 19 ethnic subgroups. They had different ancestors; therefore, they differ widely in appearance.

Where they don't differ, for the most part, is in their lifestyle and habits. Indeed, some Orang Asli continue to live in the jungles and forests as subsistence farmers, following traditional customs and practices. As with other aboriginal peoples, the Orang Asli see the land as a living entity: endowed with power and character, nature is respected, feared, appeased and lived from. Simultaneously a source of danger and a source of healing, the natural environment provides both protection and pitfalls in the form of poisonous animals, plants and disease.

Previous pages An Orang Asli settlement in Pahang, Malaysia.

Opposite The Orang Asli or 'original people' comprise 19 ethnic subgroups.

The Land and its Healing Properties

To the Orang Asli, the land is imbued with myths and magic as well as succor and shelter. It's no surprise to find there are many wonderful Orang Asli legends and tales about nature and the related origins of life. Combined with a deep knowledge and respect for plant life and the environment is a profound cultural tie to the healing traditions of their ancestors. An example of this respect is seen in early accounts of indigenous peoples' methods of harvesting plants for medicine: they would sing a little song to appease the soul or life force of the plant, to apologize for taking its life, explaining that this was to treat the suffering of a human being. While picking the plant, the gatherer would act out a ritual of hurting, articulating the sound 'ouch, ouch, ouch' in empathy with the experience of the plant itself.

This ritual illustrates how the Orang Asli are also a cultural force for conservation. They believe that only enough of a plant should be plucked, with plenty left behind for regeneration.

As in many traditional societies, Orang Asli elders are given respect and precedence; in matters of morality, spirituality, family, illness and health, they have extensive knowledge. They are both herbalists and teachers, passing on prescriptions and remedies that they, themselves, received from their elders. Believing that the forest is communal, they do not charge for their services, but freely share prescriptions for stomach ailments and headaches, wounds, bites, broken bones and allergies. Tonics, poultices, lotions and juices—taken both internally and externally—are made from barks, roots, leaves and more.

Below An Orang Asli man harvesting edible ginger roots in Taman Negara National Park, Pahang.

Opposite An old Semai woman sits with a group of young Semai children, watching their kinfolk work in the fields at the Bharat Tea Plantation in Pahang.

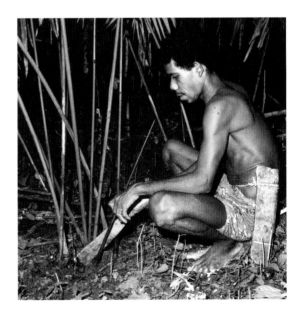

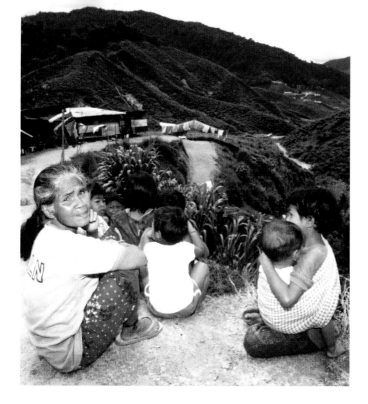

Semai Health Traditions

The Semai tribe—scattered in the regions of Middle Perak, South Perak and West Pahang—are one of the largest of the Orang Asli populations. In the past, as animists, the Semai believed that diseases were passed to humans by spirits, ghosts and demons, but, these days, they tend to accept the existence of germs. Prescriptions, however, are usually traditional—with methods and formulations taken from age-old practices.

The Semai see four important elements in life: air, fire, water and earth. They believe in the concept that air is important to all living things; thus, fire or heat plays a role in the warming up of bodies and in cooking. The water element ensures the continuity of life, while the earth (soil/land) is essential for shelter. Breathing in aroma-therapeutic air from the surrounding trees in the early morning is believed to prolong life spans and feasting the eyes on the greenery all around is a therapy in itself. Sounds heard in the night from the surrounding jungles are also thought to be able to cure illness. Finally, the Semai see that when all things die, they return to the earth.

Orang Asli elders are both herbalists and teachers, passing on prescriptions and remedies that they, themselves, received from their elders.

Sabah and Sarawak: Botanical Bounty from Borneo

As most people know, Malaysia stretches across two landmasses, each with ancient rainforests and a rich cultural heritage. While Peninsular Malaysia extends down from the Southeast Asian landmass, Borneo—across the South China Sea—is a vast island and home to the Malaysian states of Sabah and Sarawak. Containing one of the world's most complex and luxuriant rainforests, the topography ranges from interior dipterocarp forest found up to 1,200 meters above sea level, to alluvial plains and riverine forests in the lowlands.

Because of the remarkable diversity of the geography— swampy coastal lands, huge rivers, impenetrable jungles and precipitous mountains— indigenous communities tended to live in their own domains in the past. Today, a conscious effort to evolve a national culture has resulted in more integrated societies, yet each group still retains a strong ethnic, cultural and social identity.

Sabah

Sabah is Malaysia's second largest state, with an estimated population of three and a half million people. The indigenous population is made up of more than 30 groups, with the Dusun (or Kadazan-Dusun) being the largest ethnic group. Comprising about a third of the entire population, they are traditionally farmers and fishermen, with an ancient reliance on plants used as natural medicines.

A survey in 1999 of medicinal plant knowledge among the Dusun Tobilung of Kampung Toburon in Kota Belud found that all of the informants had acquired knowledge of traditional medicinal plants from another family member. While the younger generation was reported to be moving away from traditional medicine to modern medicine, there was still widespread usage and knowledge of traditional cures.

For example, the plant known to the Dusun as *sojar* or *konsuma*, to the Malays as *pokok kapal terbang*

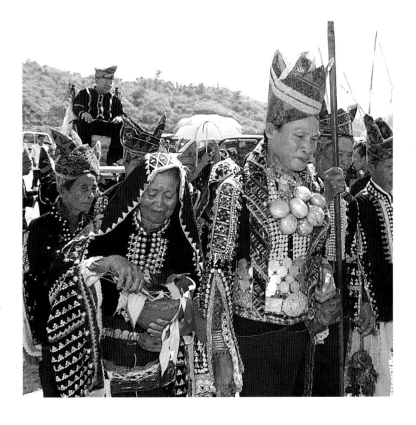

Right Kadazan-Dusun community.

Opposite Aerial view of a coastal area in Sabah, illustrating the mixed farming and fishing environments of coastal dwellers.

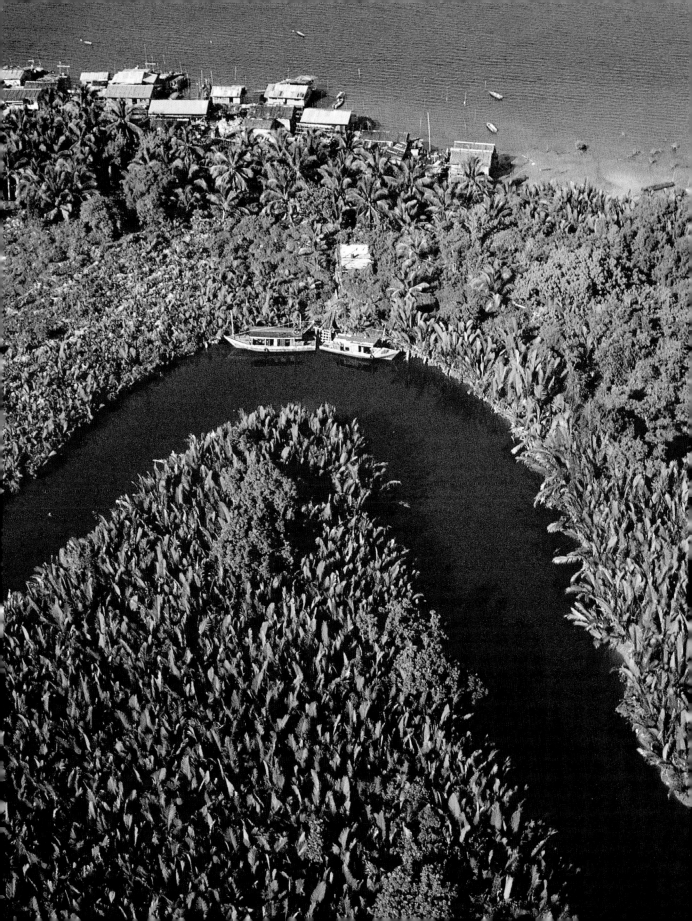

and to science as *Chromolaena odorata* is still widely used as a poultice to help with wound healing. On application, wounds are found to heal quickly with minimal scarring. Studies now back up the Dusun's claims: the plant enhances circulation in the micro-vessels of the skin, stimulates the growth of new sub-layers of the skin known as granulation tissue and promotes re-growth of the epithelium—the inner and outer layers of the skin.

Sarawak

The largest state in Malaysia, Sarawak is home to over 2 million people, three quarters of whom belong to 20 different indigenous groups. The main indigenous peoples are the Iban, the Melanau, the Bidayuh and Orang Ulu or 'people of the interior'. The Iban, who live primarily along the river systems, have traditionally held a deep spiritual connection with the rainforests they have inhabited; the Melanau tend to live in settlements along the coast and estuary of the Rejang River; the Bidayuh, comprising several distinct subgroups, live mainly in the hilly areas outside Kuching; and the Orang Ulu, as their name suggests, inhabit the interior and upland part of the country.

As with traditional societies worldwide, the forces of modernization draw young people to urban centers for employment and the encroachment of commercial farming and logging cuts deep into traditional environments. Nevertheless, there is also a natural rainforest conservation ethic among the communities of Sarawak, sometimes referred to collectively as the Dayak.

The Iban, for instance, firmly believe that forest plants have individual identities, so should not be harmed. As with other tribes, healers ask permission of plants before plucking them. Such sensitivity and respect for the essence of rainforest life inevitably places

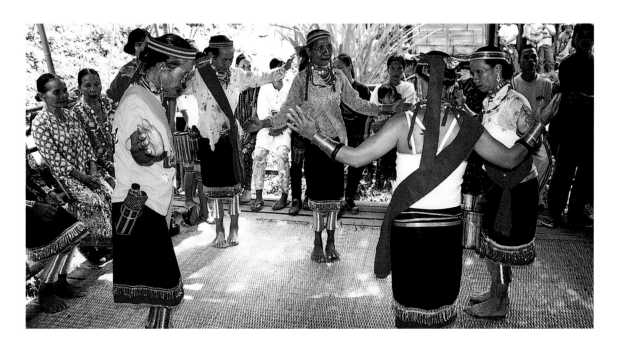

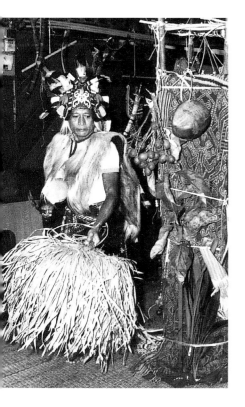

The sago palm is used extensively in healing practices among the Melanau. The cultivation of *Metroxylon sagus*, intricately linked with Melanau life for the production of sago starch, is a food attributed with varied medicinal, life-giving and even divine properties. The trunk is carved for healing ceremonies, and the fruit is given as an offering to the healing forces of nature. Unfortunately, there has been relatively little scientific research into the properties of such medicinal plants used by these rainforest communities, but it is hoped that in the future the healing potential of these plants will be further explored.

Opposite Bidayuh women, with their arms and legs adorned with brass coils, perform a ritual dance.

Above left An Iban man conducting rites during the Gawai Kenyalang festival.

Right Sago palms being harvested in Sabah.

Below Sago pith preparation.

Sarawak's indigenous communities in painful juxtaposition with the modern forces of logging and plantations, so widespread in Borneo.

Forest department research indicates greater levels of medicinal plant usage according to the degree of forest living and livelihood of the different ethnic communities of Sarawak. While the urban Chinese populations were found to use 57 local species of plants, the coastal-dwelling Melanau use 213 species, the Bidayuh use 266, the Iban use 297, and the Orang Ulu use 387.

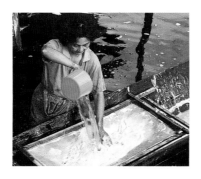

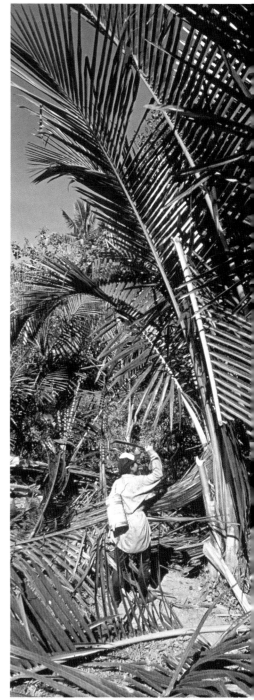

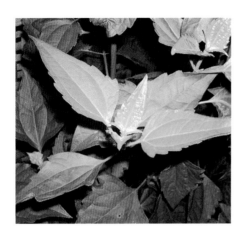

As a result, remedies for both prevention and cure of diseases from the Semai, and other Orang Asli, draw directly from the natural pharmacy that surrounds their daily lives. Recipes for common childhood ailments, pregnancy and post-natal care for women, tonics for vigor and vitality for men, and poultices and oils to ease the aches and pains of old age are all concocted from easy-to-find plants. For example, *lalang* roots (a common tall grass, *Imperata cylindrica*) are boiled and the water used to bathe children infected with jaundice; the leaves of *rumput bola* (*Hyptis rhomboidea* Mart.) are applied to sprained or twisted joints as they're believed to clear away 'dampness' and reduce swelling; vapor produced by burning the stems of *pokok kapal terbang* (*Chromolaena odorata* L.) is used to ease congestion in nasal passages; guava leaves are chewed to help with upset stomachs or to de-worm children . . . The list goes on and on.

Even the extremely common wild banana tree (*Musa acuminata*) has multifarious uses. A traditional treatment to cool down a fevered child suffering from an aching body involves immersing a piece of banana trunk in water, then dripping the water over the child's entire body. Furthermore, all parts of the banana are believed to be useful as a febrifuge and as an antidote to certain diseases, including throat infections, coughs and tonsillitis. It is also used to stop bleeding in traumatic injuries.

Above *Pokok kapal terbang* is used to ease nasal congestion.

Below Guava leaves are useful in treating upset stomachs.

Opposite Wild banana.

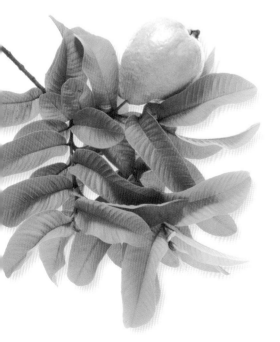

Semelai Health Traditions

The Semelai, another Orang Asli tribe, are known to have inhabited the land for more than 4000 years. Most of their villages are found in the wetlands surrounding Lake Bera in southwest Pahang; they are known to have vast knowledge of plants and their properties.

As with the Semai, the Semelai use many local plants to cure simple as well as serious diseases. The majority of cures relate to stomach complaints (*nylih ruand*) and skin ailments (*nyilih kulit*), and all parts of the plants—roots, leaves, barks— are used in cures. As with other tribal groups, there are a variety of decoctions, pastes, steams and more.

Field research in the 1970s revealed that the Semelai see plants, in many respects, in the same manner as human beings. Those plants that heal are personalized and called *puyang*. They are presumed to have souls, as do humans; one indication of this is their liquid sap is thought of as their *maham* or blood. Such plants are therefore treated with great respect, and only a small amount of any one plant is used at a time, thereby allowing that plant to continue to regenerate and grow.

Common cures for ailments are too numerous to list, but a few examples give the general idea of Semelai traditional medicine. *Vitex pubescens*, a tree sometimes cultivated for charcoal production, is used by the Semelai for minor stomachaches. The bark is stripped from the tree, boiled until it tastes bitter, then the liquid is left to cool. It is taken two to three times a day in small amounts. Another bark used, this time to help with diarrhea and dysentery, is that of *Cinnamomum verum*. This time, the bark is scraped smooth, then boiled and drunk while still quite hot. Sores are treated with a type of wild rubber of the *Willughbeia* species: shoots are chopped into fine pieces and mixed with the root sap until a type of paste forms. This is spread over sores to help them to dry up.

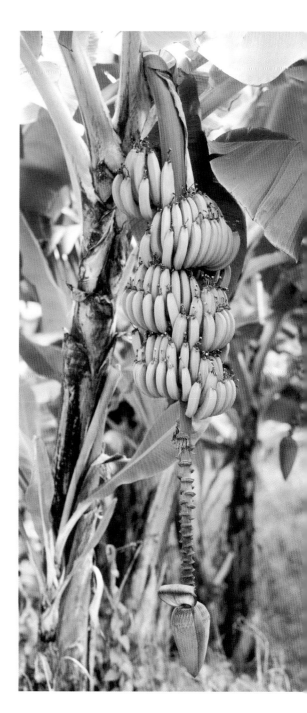

The World's Largest Flower

With more than 20 species recorded to date (although at least three are believed to be extinct), the rafflesia (*Rafflesia* spp.) is a remarkable flower. Native to Sabah in East Malaysia, Peninsular Malaysia, Sumatra, Java and the Philippines, the rafflesia is renowned not only for its flower bud which is the size of a small cabbage, but also because the flower is the only part of the plant that is visible. This is because the plant doesn't have any leaves, stems or roots as such; rather, it is a parasite, its host being a vine belonging to the *Tetrastigma* genus.

The structure of the rafflesia flower is common to all species.

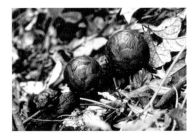

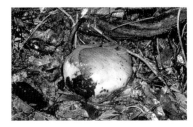

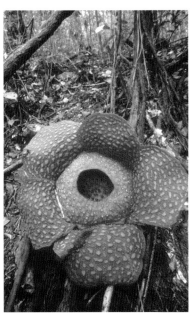

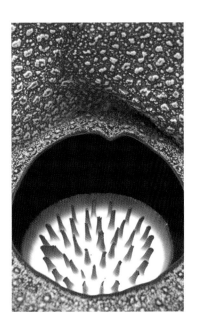

Large and round, with five fleshy lobes, the equivalent of petals, it is red in color. The largest, *R. arnoldii*, can have a diameter of up to 80 centimeters and a weight of up to seven kilograms. The flower often produces a putrid smell that attracts bluebottle flies, its primary pollinator.

The rafflesia was well known to the Orang Asli long before the 19th century when it was 'discovered' by the indefatigable Stamford Raffles in 1818. Known as *bunga pakma* or *bunga padma* in Malay (padma means lotus), it was used by the Sakai aboriginals in childbirth rituals. Taking the bud and drying it in small pieces, it was then made into a decoction. This was

believed to expedite delivery, and as it has astringent properties, it was thought to clean the uterus after childbirth. It was also believed to help the abdomen regain its shape post-natally. In the past, rafflesia extract was commonly used by men as a stimulant, while women took a rafflesia decoction as an aphrodisiac.

Even though there has been little research and no clinical studies to date, it is known that the flowers of *Rafflesia hasseltii* have anti-microbial and anti-fungal properties. Its extract is useful against certain microorganisms including some *Bacillus* and *Staphylococcus* bacteria. This goes some way to explaining its usefulness to the Orang Asli of old.

In addition to such remedies, there are specific decoctions for aiding childbirth and women in confinement and women with conditions such as ovarian cysts or amenorrhea. Overall, the Semelai medicinal traditions are quite comprehensive. Interestingly, there is some overlap with Semai traditions. For example, lalang roots (used by Semai in the treatment of jaundice) are used by the Semelai as a remedy for coughs and colds. After cleaning the roots to remove any itchy powdery substances caught in them, they are boiled and the ensuing sweet decoction is taken to soothe a persistent cough.

Age-old Wisdoms, Future Practices

Over the centuries, many of these traditional practices have been adopted and adapted by Malay populations, and, time and again, we see the same plants and herbs used in both cultures. However, certain remedies remain ensconced in the domain of the Orang Asli, jealously guarded and protected for posterity. Unfortunately, partly because of this secrecy, partly because many Orang Asli remedies are undocumented, and certainly because of the degradation of their environments, there is a real danger that their knowledge is fast disappearing.

The recent interest by other countries in plant-based medicines has led to more research into such age-old wisdoms. This is certainly desirable, but needs to be handled with care. However, if the global thirst for more natural solutions to health problems results in some Orang Asli traditions being preserved for posterity, it is so much the better. There's no doubt that their ancient apothecary holds, if not the elixir of life, plenty of life-enhancing formulae that can be further developed in the future.

Opposite, clockwise from top right
A rafflesia flower at Gunung Gading National Park, Borneo; a close-up of the rafflesia; buds of the parasitic plant *Rafflesia tuan-mudae* blooming in lowland rainforest; buds of the *Rafflesia keithii* near Mount Kinabalu National Park, Sabah.

Traditional Asli Jakun Medicinal Heritage Garden: A UNDP/GEF Project

The United Nations Development Programme (UNDP) and the Global Environment Facility (GEF) run a number of development projects in Malaysia, one of which is located in the state of Pahang at Kampung Simpai within an Orang Asli reserve. Home to about 1,300 people of the Asli Jakun, an Orang Asli subgroup, the project is aimed at conserving their traditional resources. The livelihood and medical needs of this community depend on resources from a nearby peat swamp forest, which, due to logging, commercial agriculture and forest fires, is dwindling.

Collaboration with the village committee resulted in the following objectives being agreed upon:
1. Cultivate medicinal and other related plants of importance to the Jakun community.
2. Preserve traditional knowledge through the publication of a booklet on the indigenous knowledge of the Asli Jakun.
3. Provide a supplementary livelihood to the local community, in particular by supplying raw materials to women handicraft makers.

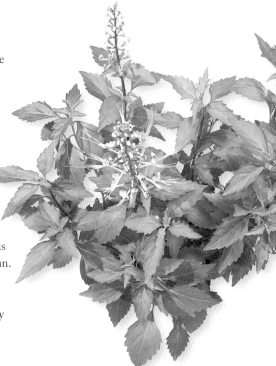

4. Forge collaboration with the scientific community and establish a benefits-sharing mechanism.

Five hectares of land within the Orang Asli reserve—part peat swamp and part lowland dipterocarp forest—were allocated for the preservation and planting of various medicinal plants. A nursery was set up both to cultivate plants and generate raw materials to be used by the handicraft makers. With the involvement of a number of agencies, including indigenous

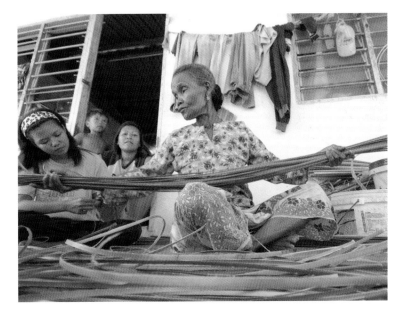

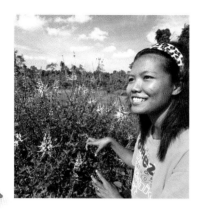

NGOs, some of the youths were trained to implement the project, while the UNDP provided financial support. A leading research institute in Malaysia did soil studies and a cost benefit analysis, and then trained community members on the planting and cultivation of *misai kucing* (*Orthosiphon stamineus*), *pegaga* (*Centella asiatica*) and *bunga melur* (*Jasminum sambac*). The institute also organized the collection of herbarium samples for recording and documentation.

The Jakun community worked with other local and regional indigenous organizations such as Partners of Community Organizations (PACOS) and a Philippine-based international organization on indigenous rights. Despite many challenges, there were some positive impacts, particularly as regards the high level of awareness and interest among community members to respect and record their indigenous knowledge. Also, the youth and older community members worked together to create a network of indigenous support for the Jakun community and facilitate the formulation of a Heritage Garden Protocol Statement.

Projects such as these further the protection and conservation of traditional knowledge and are to be encouraged. In the long term, they will also help with Malaysia's plans to globalize its herbal healing traditions and practices.

Opposite, above A *misai kucing* plant.

Opposite, below The UNDP/ GEF development project aims to conserve the Asli Jakun's traditional resources.

Clockwise from top left A young Asli Jakun lady shows off a *misai kucing* shrub, one of many plants cultivated under the UNDP/ GEF project; a *bunga melur* plant; *pegaga* plants.

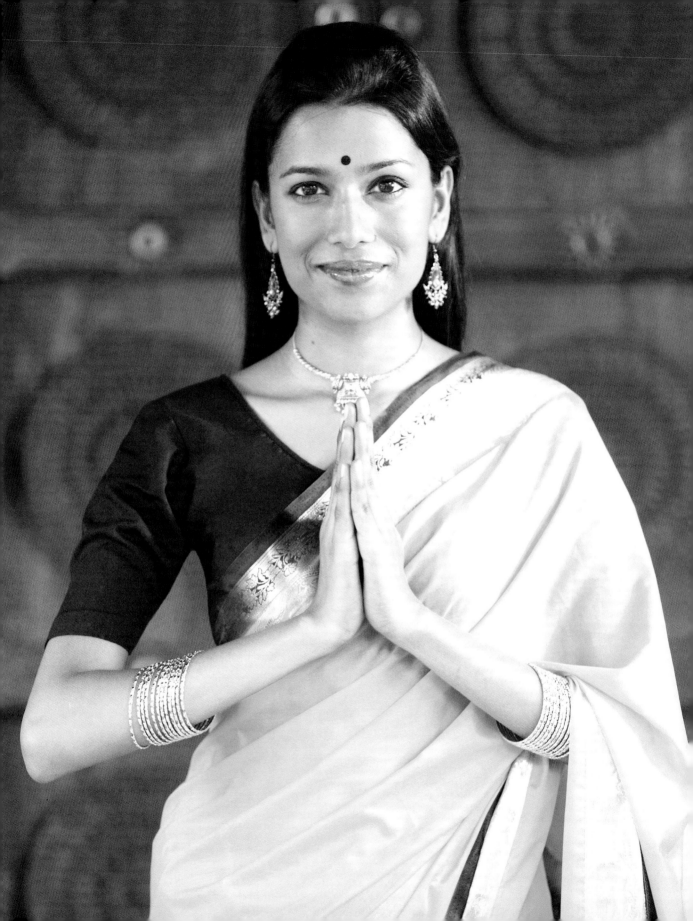

Indian Health Traditions
From the Vedas to Modern-Day Malaysia

The ancient system of healing known as Ayurveda, which means the 'science of life', has been, and still is, gaining popularity worldwide. Ayurveda places emphasis on caring for one's health by nurturing body, mind and spirit, and taking time to heal and grow. This age-old tradition encompasses treatments from the *abhyanga* body massage to *sirodhara*, in which oil is poured in a continuous stream onto the forehead of the patient.

Such an approach to health, wellbeing and beauty resonates with everyone, especially in a world that is increasingly hectic and stressful. The concept of practicing self-healing by using oils, herbs and a balanced diet are part of this ancient tradition. Ayurveda takes into account the need for inner development, and involves not only physical conditions, but mental and emotional ones too. Indeed, Ayurveda, which has been in existence for 5,000 years, is still relevant today.

India has other medical disciplines as well. Siddha, Unani, the practices of yoga for health, *pranayama* and meditation for tranquility and inner development, as well as a host of home-care regimes are regularly practiced for general wellbeing. Although these disciplines all have unique theories and practices, they share similarities with Ayurveda—they are all unified in their desire to live in harmony with the natural world. In addition, for the most part, they employ only natural remedies.

Opposite Ayurveda seeks to achieve balance in one's physical, mental, spiritual and emotional conditions.

As we've seen, local Malay healthcare traditions embody many of these ideas as well. But how did they come to be influenced by Indian systems?

Indians in the Malay Peninsula

Imagine an ancient civilized city, with soaring temples, palaces, civic buildings and centers of learning. Founded in the 1st century CE by Tamil dynasties of southern India, this civilization was situated on the west coast of the Malay Peninsula. According to early Tamil and Chinese records, it was easily accessible from south India's Coromandel Coast and was a place of great felicity and abundance. An important outpost on the ancient Spice Route, it had a flourishing social and economic life. Its Sanskrit name was Suvarnabhumi or 'the place of golden earth', but most knew it by the Tamil name of Kadaram (known as Kedah today). Home at different times to major religious centers of Hinduism and Buddhism, it was a hub for silk and jewelry production, metallurgy and religious sculpture, and for learning.

Archeological excavations in an area known as the Bujang Valley in southern Kedah have revealed ancient temples or *candi*, a host of temple artifacts, jewelry, gold ornaments, and fine stone and bronze statues. The structural design and orientation of the candi, as well as their decorative features, are evidence of influences from principles of ancient Vedic architecture, or *vastu*. The Vedic sciences include advanced systems of design, astronomy, medicine, plant science, physics, metallurgy and many others. Now proposed for UNESCO listing as an archeological park, the Bujang Valley holds great promise of revealing much more about ancient Indian influences on the Malay Peninsula.

Formerly known as Suvarnabhumi ('the Place of the Golden Earth') in Sanskrit, Kedah was home at different times to major religious centers of Hinduism and Buddhism.

Amalaka—An Ayurvedic Wonder Fruit

The fruit of the Indian gooseberry (*Emblica officinalis*) is one of the most important ingredients in Ayurvedic medicine. It is used widely as a tonic, immune system booster and as a means of promoting youthful vigor. One of the three ingredients that make up *triphala* powder—an Ayurvedic formulation used as a laxative and for headaches, biliousness, dyspepsia, constipation, piles and enlarged liver—Indian gooseberry is considered an Ayurvedic wonder plant. Known as *amla*, *amala*, *amlaka* and *amlika* in India, its Malay name is very similar—*amalaka* or amla.

This nomenclature has an interesting aside in modern Malaysia's history, generally considered to have begun with the emergence of the Melaka Sultanate in the 15th century. When the roving Palembang prince Parameswara first set foot at the small fishing village of Melaka, he was taken with it and saw it as a possible future kingdom. On asking the locals the name for the tree under which he and his retinue were seated, the answer Parameswara received was 'amalaka'.

This was the name the prince gave to his new kingdom, a name that later became abbreviated from Amalaka to Melaka. Of course, nobody at the time could have foreseen how such an innocent tree could have had such widespread influence, firstly in the Malay Peninsula, then in the wider world with the emergence of the Straits Settlements and the massive trade that came with it. Even today, Melaka is a bustling small city, rich in culture, architecture and tradition. Interestingly, in Indian health traditions, amalaka's uses are as diverse and plentiful as is the reach and influence of the great trading port and Straits named after it.

The fruit of the amalaka tree—native to Malaysia, India, Sri Lanka and China—is a highly concentrated source of vitamin C and is rich in calcium, phosphorus and iron. Amalaka's ascorbic acid content, ranging from 1,100 to 1,700 milligrams per 100 grams, is reportedly the second highest of all fruits, second only to the Barbados cherry and higher than the fabled blueberry! Recent research in India has revealed that amalaka has powerful antioxidant properties and may have anti-cancer properties too. More studies are currently underway.

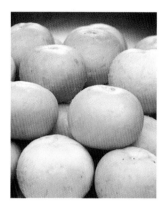

Above Amala fruit.

Below A painting depicting Parameswara in Melaka.

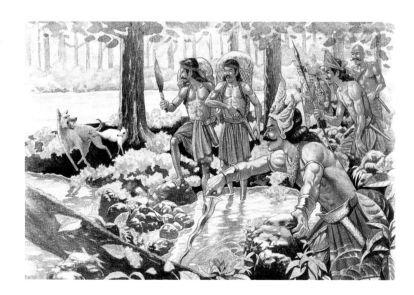

Taking its name from 18 Tamil *siddhars* (those who attained *siddhi* or perfection), the Siddha medical system shares with Ayurveda the theory of five elements and three *doshas*, which are referred to as *muppini* in Tamil.

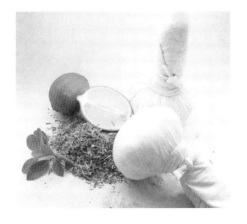

Indian Medical Traditions

Ayurveda is the most widely practiced of India's medical systems and, like the wider system of India's Vedic science, it begins with a theory grounded in the five basic elements of creation. Known as *panchamahabhuta*—*panch* means five, *maha* means great and *bhuta* means elements—these elements are earth, fire, water, air and space. Ayurveda also identifies three basic principles of physiology known as *doshas*, which emerge from these five elements. They are motion, metabolism and structure. Motion is characterized by the wind element or *vata*; metabolism by fire or *pitta*; and structure by water or *kapha*.

From this broad theory, Ayurveda goes on to describe categories of human physiology, types of diseases resulting from unbalanced doshas, treatments to restore balance, and general advice on diet, lifestyle habits and more. In essence, Ayurveda provides a framework for daily life, offering insights into how best to live attuned to the cycles of the day and the rhythms of the seasons.

Greatly similar to Ayurveda is the Tamil medical system known as Siddha. Taking its name from 18 Tamil *siddhars* (devotees of Shiva who attained *siddhi* or perfection), it shares with Ayurveda the theory of five elements and three doshas, which are referred to as *muppini* in Tamil. However, unlike Ayurveda, Siddha divides the body according to the five elements. So, earth corresponds to the legs, water to the abdomen, fire to the chest, air to the neck and space to the head. It also relates the five elements to bodily fluids.

Alchemical ideas dominate Siddha medicine with its *materia medica* consisting of herbs, roots, salts, metals and mineral compounds. It emphasizes the importance of mineral preparations in treatment, which, although present in Ayurveda, are not given the same degree of prominence. A diet containing fresh plants is also at the forefront of Siddha, as is yoga and the philosophy of inner development.

As with Ayurveda, the pursuit of longevity without illness and a purposeful life of inner fullness is Siddha's ultimate aim.

Another medical influence that has taken root on the Malay Peninsula from India is Unani medicine. It originated in Greece and was founded by the philosopher-physician Hippocrates (460–377 BCE) and was formulated over time by various Islamic scholar physicians in what is now the Middle East. It was introduced to India during the medieval period, but grew in influence under Moghul patronage. With the growth of Islam in the Malay Peninsula and neighboring countries, Unani medicine spread even further.

Unani medicine is based on the humoral theory, which is the presence and balance of blood, phlegm, yellow and black bile, and remedies are generally herb-based. Over time, aspects of Islam were introduced to its Greco-Arabic theory; one example of this is an emphasis on the healing aspects of honey, which draws from Qur'anic recommendations and spiritual approaches to healing.

Even though Unani differs in many ways from Malay medicine, some aspects have been absorbed into Malay health practices. This is particularly the case in the humoral theory of both. It's also interesting to see how many Malay herbal remedies have parallels with both Ayurvedic and Siddha formulations.

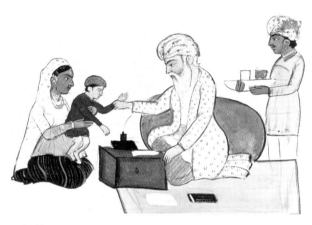

Opposite Siddha medicine, from the ancient Tamil traditions of India, uses fresh ingredients in many of its preparations.

Above A 19th-century Indian painting depicting a Unani practitioner examining a patient.

Below Hippocrates (460–377 BCE).

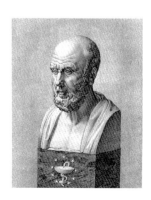

The Bujang Valley Civilization

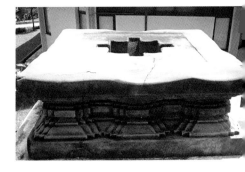

Archeologists are still working on the vast 224 square kilometer region that makes up the Bujang Valley historical complex. Yet, it is clear that the area, located in the state of Kedah, is among the oldest and richest in Malaysia.

Archeological research has established that an ancient Hindu-Buddhist civilization once flourished here at least 1,500 years ago. Up to the present time, a series of ancient temples called *candi* have been excavated, the most impressive being found in Pengkalan Bayan Merobok, where the Bujang Valley's archeological museum is also located.

The Bujang Valley area of Kedah, known in ancient Tamil as Kadaram,

was probably the earliest and most important landfall for South Indian traders from Tamil Nadu, especially during the reign of the Pallava Kings between the 4th and 9th centuries CE. As it was geographically positioned on the same latitude as southern India, it allowed ships to sail due east or due west through the Bay of Bengal without getting lost. Equally, Chinese ships coming to trade with the West or to bring pilgrims to Buddhist holy sites in India, found Kadaram an ideal and felicitous port to rest and replenish supplies.

The sight of Gunung Jerai's peak, looming high above the horizon, lit by a beacon of light from

a permanently blazing pyre, must have been a welcome sight, guiding these early sailors. Isolated from the other mountain ranges of Peninsular Malaysia, its slopes contain a unique range of medicinal plants and herbs not found in other areas of Malaysia, surely testament to its early settlers.

Trading relations between India and the Malay Peninsula led to the gradual indigenization of

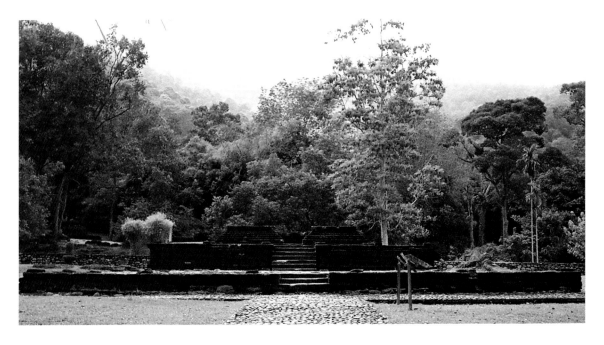

Indian culture on parts of the Malay Peninsular coast, especially with Kadaram on the west coast and its counterpart civilization, Langkasuka, on Malaysia's northeast coast.

During the 11th century, these cultural and commercial ties were reinforced when India's Chola monarch, Rajendra I, extended his influence as far eastwards as the Srivijayan ports of Sumatra, including, it would seem, Kedah and the Bujang Valley.

Besides the ancient candi, mostly collapsed but now gradually undergoing restoration, the Bujang Valley Archaeological Museum contains stone caskets clearly inscribed in South Indian scripts, Hindu iconography and an impressive collection of early ceramics and pottery. There is a Sanskrit inscription dating from the 4th century CE, discovered in the mid-19th century by a certain Captain James Low, along with a slab

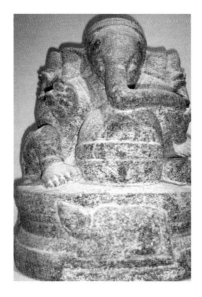

found in the estuary of the Muda River that bears a Sanskrit prayer in 5th-century Pallava script. The message on the slab wishes for the success of a voyage about to be undertaken by a sailing master, thus indicating that Kedah was a home port to Indian traders from very early times.

Chinese diary entries from a century or so later describe a Buddhist pilgrim's delight with Kadaram as a place of 'great felicity', of silk production and the manufacture of fine jewelry and gold ornaments, and of cultured living and the arts.

From this, it is apparent that Kedah provided the earliest and most important link yet discovered between Southern and Eastern Asia and the Malay world. It also partially explains the enduring influence of so many Indian customs, practices and linguistic roots in contemporary Malay culture.

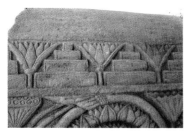

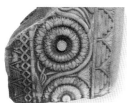

Opposite, top The marks of centuries of veneration worn into its ancient steps, this statue-base would have formed a central feature in a *candi* in ancient Kadaram.

Opposite, bottom The base of a *candi* situated on Gunung Jerai in Kedah. For centuries, a large fire was maintained on the mountain, day and night, serving the dual purpose of a beacon for ships sailing into the safe harbor of Kadaram and as a sacred fire representing the religious traditions of the region.

Left This very early Ganesh statue indicates the Shaivite traditions of ancient Kadaram.

Below left Lotus blossoms adorn the four tiered *candi* carved into pink stone—possibly part of a doorway or altarpiece in one of the many candis of Kadaram.

Below A temple ornament—possibly a guardian figure—now housed in the Lembah Bujang Museum on Gunung Jerai.

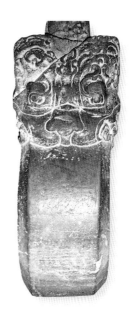

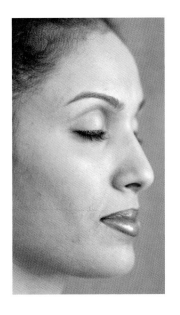

Ayurveda and Home Beauty Care

According to Ayurvedic texts, the basis for beauty is a substance called *ojas*, a refined product that literally means 'vigor' in Sanskrit. Ojas also refers to a subtle and vital fluid that Ayurveda holds is produced via digestion and is itself the finest product of digestion. It is described as the essence of the body tissues or *dhatus*, indicating that a healthy digestion and fresh food form the basis for radiant skin. Indeed, in Ayurveda, there is an expression that 'without proper diet medicine is of no use, while with proper diet medicine is of no need'.

Indian families following Ayurvedic traditions in Malaysia have taken this saying to heart. Their habit of a balanced, largely vegetarian diet, modified according to season and the *doshic* needs of different family members, is part and parcel of their daily routine or *dinacharya*. But even though they follow Ayurvedic medicine and cooking principles, they also introduce local Malay ingredients into the mix. For example, the well-known *petai* bean (*Parkia speciosa*), sometimes rudely known as the stink bean due to its pungent smell, is used in Ayurveda for urinary control, cleansing of the kidneys, and as a kidney tonic. It is also used in Malay food-medicine.

In addition to diet, many Malaysian Indian women follow the *doshic* theory of skincare that identifies three basic skin types—vata, pitta and kapha—with which unique treatments are matched. Following the specific recommendations results in a radiant and clear complexion.

Ayurvedic texts describe vata dosha as having the characteristics of light, dry and cool. Therefore, vata-type skin is typically thin, delicate and dry, with fine pores. It feels cool to the touch. With age, it is prone to wrinkling due to its intrinsic dryness and, when unbalanced, it tends to be dry, rough or

Above The doshic theory of skincare identifies three basic skin types—*vata*, *pitta* and *kapha*.

Below The *petai* bean is believed to cleanse the kidneys.

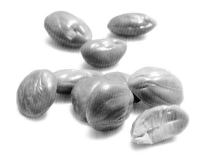

Ayurvedic Herbs for Common Childhood Ailments

Even though many local recipes for common childhood ailments have been adopted by Indians who settled in the Malay Peninsula, there are quite a few prescriptions unique to Indian households. Drawing on Ayurvedic roots, Indians have taken local herbs readily available in Malaysia to substitute for those used by their forefathers in India. Indeed, Malaysia's rich rainforest bestows bounty far and wide.

In the case of jaundice, Indian mothers often recommend *Phyllanthus niruri* leaves and roots boiled with goat's milk. Commonly known as 'stonebreaker' because of its strong roots, all parts of the plant are used in Ayurvedic medicine, as it is well known for its diuretic, analgesic, anti-spasmodic, febrifugal and cell protective properties. As it is a common weed, it is easily harvested.

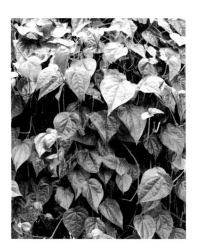

Betel leaves (*Piper betle*), when mixed with pure coconut oil and fresh turmeric juice, are commonly used to treat areas of inflammation. The leaves are first slightly warmed, then applied onto the inflamed area a few times. If a baby has colic, betel leaves are smeared with castor oil and toasted over a flame and, while still warm, are placed over the abdomen to encourage the baby to expel wind.

Turmeric (*Curcuma longa*), the Ayurvedic wonder rhizome found in countless herbal healing recipes, finds its way into many concoctions for both children and adults. For diarrhea, a teaspoonful of fresh turmeric is mixed with the juice extracted from the holy basil plant (*Ocimum tenuiflorum*) and given once every four hours until symptoms clear up.

And as a beautifier, vetiver roots (*Chrysopogon zizanioides*) are dried and crushed into a powder and added to *Curcuma aromatica* rhizome and Indian gooseberry fruit (*Emblica officinalis*), both also dried and ground into a powder. These are mixed with the petals of dried rose (for its sweet scent) and used as a complexion booster. It makes a useful mask to treat pimples and dark pigmentation on the face and also finds itself in adult facials to enhance radiance. It is used on the skin of children to smoothen the complexion and boost skin health.

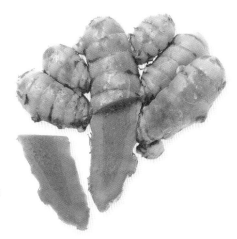

Clockwise from top Fresh turmeric; vetiver roots; betel leaves.

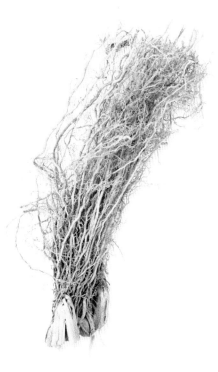

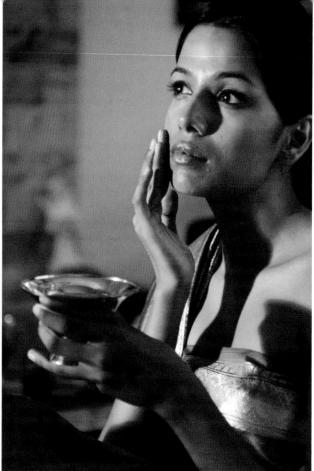

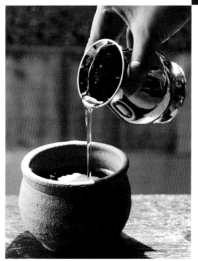

flaky. It can also exhibit dry forms of eczema and fungus. Vata skin is also a mirror for mental stress and takes on a tired, stressed and even grayish look. With this dryness, moisture is the key to retaining beauty of fine vata skin, so oils, creams and oil baths are central to vata skin health.

Pitta-type skin, on the other hand, is warmer, softer, rosier and thicker than vata skin. Rosacea (rashes, acne, liver spots and redness in the middle part of the face) is an indicator of unbalanced pitta. The key to managing pitta skin is to avoid direct sunlight. Here, the UV-protectant effect of oils, such as cold-pressed coconut oil, have protected Malaysian women from the harmful ultraviolet rays of the tropical sun. A 'cooling' diet containing foods such as bitter gourd, and a regular routine with early bedtime are all common remedies for lowering the 'heat' of pitta dosha.

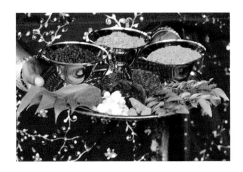

Skin that is typical of kapha dosha is thicker, softer and oilier than the other skin types. Fortunately for those with kapha skin, they are less inclined to wrinkles as they age. However, when out of balance, their skin can be excessively oily with enlarged pores, blackheads and damp forms of eczema. Regular cleansing is important for kapha-type skin, so lubricating a couple of times a week with gingelly oil (see page 200), or another nutritional oil, such as almond, is a good first step. Ayurveda considers, quite naturally, that avoiding oily and heavy foods benefits kapha-type skin.

More generally, good-quality food is of central value in creating and maintaining skin health. Stale food is believed to result in the development of toxins, known as *ama* in Ayurveda. Accumulations of ama are to be avoided at all cost as they can cause damage to the body's tissues. This is not so dissimilar to the explanations in modern medicine of the effects of oxidation causing food to spoil and oxidative stress leading to damage to arterial linings and to the body's organ systems.

The spices used in Indian cooking are also very helpful for skin health. Turmeric is a powerful anti-inflammatory agent and, in the Ayurvedic view, affects the deeper layers of tissue, including skin. Spices believed to purify the blood and cleanse fatty tissue from the body include cumin, fenugreek and black pepper as well as turmeric. Ayurveda considers that black pepper and turmeric also help cleanse the body of waste matter by excreting it through sweat, thereby creating healthier skin in the process. Many other plants are also considered beneficial for beauty; whether ingested or applied topically, such kitchen cosmetics have been grown, nurtured, plucked and used by Malaysian Indian households for centuries.

Opposite, above Those with *vata*-type skin should moisturize with oil.

Opposite, below Gingelly, or sesame, oil is a basic ingredient in many Ayurvedic treatments.

Above Dried spices such as black pepper, cumin and fenugreek from the Indian kitchen pharmacy, combine with fresh betel and neem leaf, rose, jasmine and turmeric root to create a widely available and popular range of home preparations for enhancing immunity.

Yoga and Meditation

Yoga, which means 'union' or 'to join together' in Sanskrit, is practiced in the Vedic tradition as a way of bringing together mind and body. From a health perspective, yoga and Ayurveda have the same goal—a healthy person with a balanced mind. Yoga is described in the *Yoga Sutras* of Patanjali as *yogas chitta vritti nirodhaha* or the 'settled state of mind'.

Charaka Samhita, the preeminent Ayurvedic text, mentions yoga as being helpful in removing tension, improving digestion and integrating bodily and mental functions. It is also seen as a means for calming the mind before meditation. Meditation, now proven by numerous scientific studies to reduce stress, enhances cardiovascular functioning and reduces disease severity.

From the earliest Indian presence on the Malay Peninsula, yoga has been an abiding influence. Temple sculptures excavated at the Bujang Valley portray gentle yoga positions. Today, 2,000 years later, yoga—including many schools of *hatha yoga* (the physical system), *pranayama* (the breathing system), and *dhyan* or meditation—is widely practiced in Malaysia. Recognized as a means of achieving balance and integration of mind and body, it is taught through traditional schools, families and yoga masters. The tradition has endured and is now widespread in fitness and yoga centers.

Indian Influences in Malaysian Health Traditions

A theory of elements is present in Malay medicine. Indeed, all four of the elements used in Malay medical theory—earth, fire, water and air—are almost congruent with those of

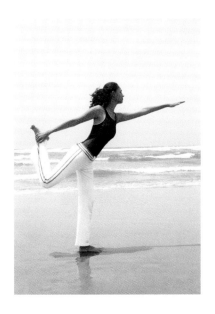

Above The 'king dancer', or *Natarajasana*, pose strengthens legs and improves balance.

Opposite Yoga is helpful in integrating bodily and mental functions.

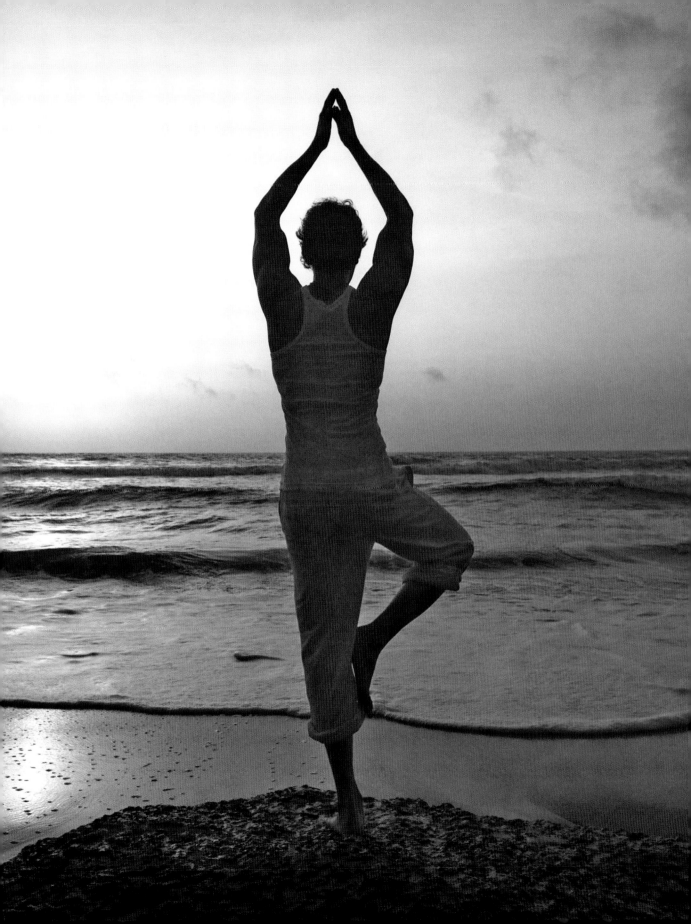

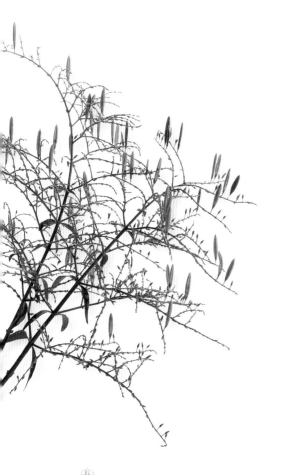

Above *Andrographis paniculata*,
known as *hempedu bumi* in Malay,
is used to reduce heat in both Malay
and Indian traditions.

Below Indian gooseberry
or *amala*.

Opposite Herbal oil massages
are part of Ayurvedic traditions.

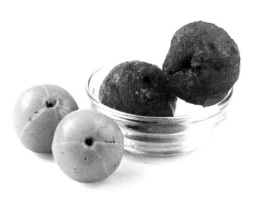

Ayurveda and Siddha. In neighboring Thailand and nearby Myanmar, both of whose medical systems derive from Ayurveda, the same theory of four elements can be found. While converging fully with Ayurvedic theory, there is also some partial overlap with TCM theory and its emphasis on the five elements of earth, fire, water, wood and metal.

Malay and Ayurvedic food recommendations and taboos for health promotion are also in parallel. The Malay classification of 'hot', 'cold' and 'gassy' foods correlates with Ayurveda's *tridosha* theory. In Malay food tradition, these are *angin* (vata or wind), *panas* (pitta or heat) and *sejuk* (kapha or cold and damp).

Similarly, Ayurvedic and Malay herbal traditions share many common plant-based medicines. The bitter herb *Andrographis paniculata*, a potent febrifuge and anti-viral agent, is used in both traditions to reduce heat. *Tinospora cordifolia*, although native to India, is found in Penang and Perak and is used for strength in Malay medicine and as a tonic in Ayurveda. The Indian gooseberry or *amala* (*Emblica officinalis*) is used by both cultures for general strength and balance. Native to Malaysia, India, Sri Lanka and China, it is a highly concentrated source of vitamin C and is rich in calcium, phosphorus and iron. Indian families often add amala to their sesame oil and use this as hair oil. Partly due to its 20 percent tannin content, it gives a lustrous dark color to the hair. Aromatic holy basil (*Ocimum tenuiflorum*) and the plant *Centella asiatica* are both used as brain tonics in Ayurveda and for similar applications in Malay medicine. The list goes on and on!

Other parallels between Malay and Ayurvedic traditions include the practices of Malay post-natal care or *berpantang*. Found throughout rural and much of urban

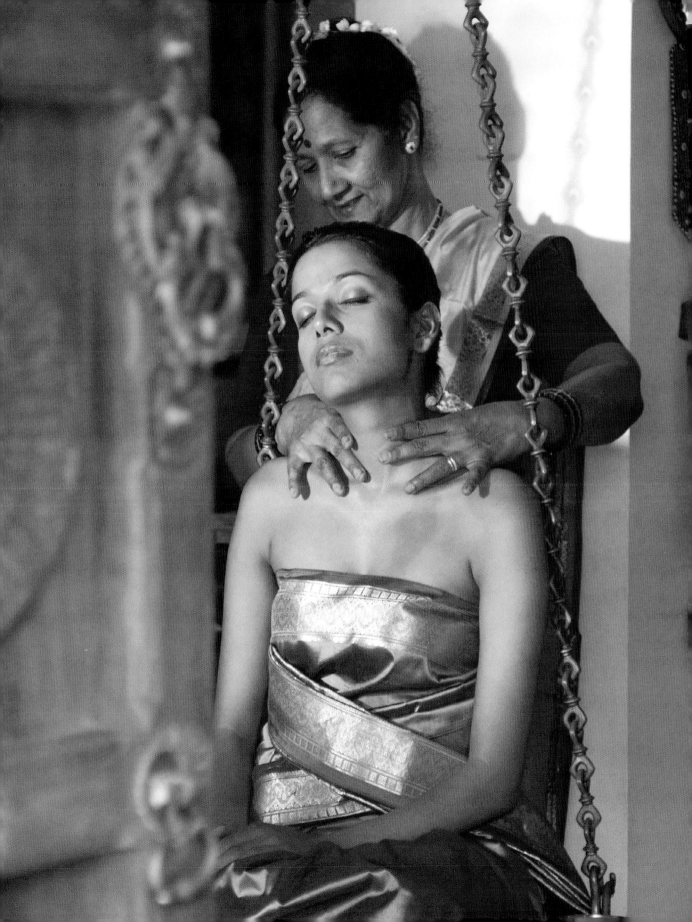

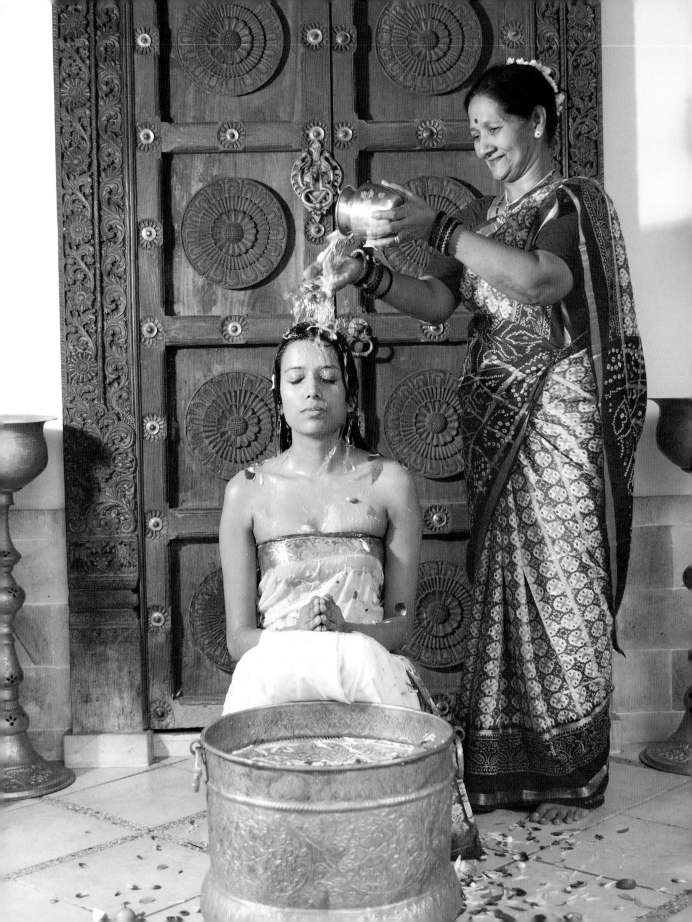

Malaysia (and increasingly popular outside Malaysia), it involves 44 days of confinement, massages using herbal oils, a unique and nourishing diet, wrapping the torso tightly with a special cloth to return the body to its pre-pregnancy shape, and treatments for vaginal and uterine health. Unsurprisingly, such a system is also found in the villages in South India. Malaysians use frankincense, the aromatic resin from *Boswellia sacra*, in their massages and south Indian midwives are known for making an oil from this plant and using it for massaging and wrapping. The practice of floral bathing for therapeutic cleansing is also found in both countries (see page 195); in fact, the exotic floral bath has now become an essential treatment in Asian-themed spas.

In the area of beauty, Malay and Ayurvedic traditions share many similarities in the practices for promoting lustrous hair, bright eyes and a clear complexion. The delicate *cempaka* flower and rice flour mask that Malaysian women apply on their faces at night to enhance the complexion has similarities with Ayurvedic cempaka uses. The jasmine flower is used for its sweet fragrance in both cultures. Indians as well as Malaysians find coconut milk a particularly effective hair conditioner. Also known as *santan*, coconut milk is an important ingredient in Malaysian cuisine and can be readily found in local markets.

Malaysia's national flower, the red hibiscus (*Hibiscus rosa-sinensis*), is also used in traditional Ayurvedic haircare. Rich in nutrients, it is used as a treatment for a range of medical conditions, including gynecological. Drawing on Indian traditions, Malaysian Indian women boil the flowers and leaves and add the essence to coconut or sesame oil for application to the hair. This lends a lustrous black sheen to naturally dark hair and is also reported to promote hair growth. In the past, women also burned the flowers and leaves to make a type

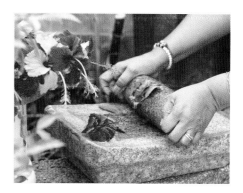

Opposite Traditional Indian floral bath.

Above Hibiscus leaves and flowers are ground before they are boiled with sesame or coconut oil.

Below The hibiscus concoction promotes lustrous and dark hair.

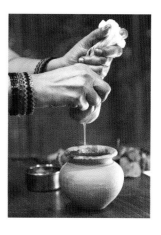

of kohl. Mixing the hibiscus ash with a type of clarified butter called ghee produces a natural dye for blackening around the eyelids and eyebrows. In addition to its cosmetic benefit, the darkening of the eyelids also provides relief from the strong glare of Malaysia's equatorial sun.

Another ingredient for keeping hair healthy and dark is *bringhraj* (*Eclipta alba*). A moisture-loving creeper with small, white flowers, it grows in abundance in the tropics. Picked and boiled to an extract by Indian mothers in Malaysia, it was added to sesame-oil hair baths to enhance hair luster and growth.

The Future

With daily wellness and beauty regimes, herbal remedies and a plethora of exotic practices, it is apparent that Indian health traditions have permeated the Malaysian way of life. Today, this is taken a step further with the emergence of Malaysian-themed spas, many of which offer unique fusions of Malay and Ayurvedic traditions often combined with wisdom and techniques from TCM. These spas promote, preserve and further blend the ancient wellness traditions of India and Malaysia.

Corresponding with this, the Malaysian government is promoting Ayurvedic programs in hospitals and the training and licensing of Ayurvedic physicians in Malaysia. Similarly, an association of practitioners of Indian traditional medicine in Malaysia is working to bring all the practitioners of these disciplines together to promote high-quality, professional standards to better serve the public. With such dedication and resolve, the future of Ayurveda, and other Indian systems, looks set to grow in Malaysia.

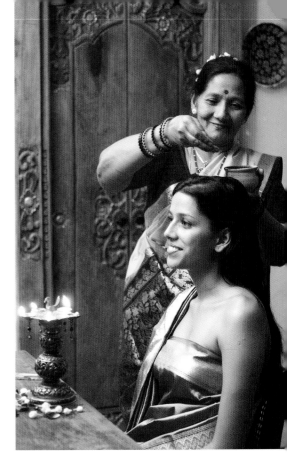

Above Sesame oil hair baths enhance hair luster and growth.

Below Golden chrysanthemum, rose, lime and jasmine blossoms—essential components for pacifying the senses.

Opposite Lime juice, honey and curry leaves are used to treat morning sickness.

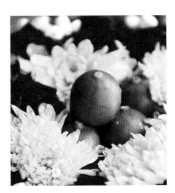

Pre- and Post-Natal Care in the Ayurvedic Tradition

Indian traditional health systems advocate total wellness during pregnancy and in the post-natal period. The mother is looked after with extreme care especially as regards her diet: many of the foods ingested daily are designed to boost the mother's immune system and give her energy; some also encourage the baby to produce strong bones and an allergy-free skin. After the baby is born, other dishes help the mother regain her strength, while special procedures are practiced to ensure the baby is healthy and strong.

Indians in Malaysia have carried on their traditional systems, sometimes substituting local herbs for those used in India. So, what are some of the herbs and what do they do?

During pregnancy, *Moringa oleifera* or drumstick tree leaves are cooked with garlic, ginger, cumin powder, turmeric powder and fenugreek seeds and given to the mother-to-be once or twice a week, and more often during the last trimester. This is because the leaves act as a galactagogue—that is, they help to stimulate the production of breast milk after delivery. They are also rich in vitamins A and C and the seeds help maintain the normal physiology of the uterus.

Morning sickness is often treated with the ubiquitous curry leaf (*Murraya koenigii*). Grown in most backyards as it is a staple in Indian cuisine, it is readily available. One teaspoonful of fresh curry leaf juice is mixed with a teaspoon of lime juice and honey to settle the stomach; it also aids the digestion as the leaves are mildly laxative.

After the birth of the baby, a different set of herbs helps the mother to recover from the stresses and strains of delivery. *Cissus quadrangularis* is cooked in a soup together with black pepper, garlic, ginger, coriander leaves and galangal rhizomes to nourish and revitalize; it is also a great anti-rheumatic, so may be taken again later in life.

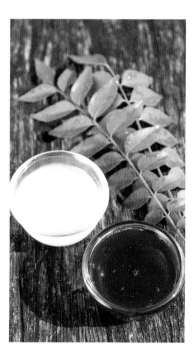

To induce a good night's sleep during the post-natal period, neem leaves (*Azadirachta indica*) and mashed turmeric rhizome are boiled in an earthen pot and the water is used to bathe the body at least twice a week from head to toe. After this, good quality frankincense is burned to smoke the feet of the mother, thereby transferring heat to the soles of the feet to strengthen nerves.

If the mother shows signs of puerperal fever (also known as childbed fever as it is frequently contracted shortly after childbirth), a decoction of *Leucas aspera* is recommended. If the fever turns into a cold, the leaves and stems are cooked into a health-giving soup with pepper, garlic, ginger, coriander and a small amount of galangal.

As with other Asian cultures, the baby is massaged—with sesame oil in the Indian tradition—at least three times a week before bathing to strengthen bones, skin and muscles. And bathwater benefits from boiled sweet basil leaves (*Ocimum basilicum*) and neem leaves: these act as an antiseptic against a wide range of common bacteria.

Indian borage (*Plectranthus amboinicus*) is another frequently used herb in the baby's early life. Used as a concoction with a few drops of honey and a drop of pure castor oil, it is an immunomodulator, clearing the baby's lungs and sinuses and expelling wind from the stomach.

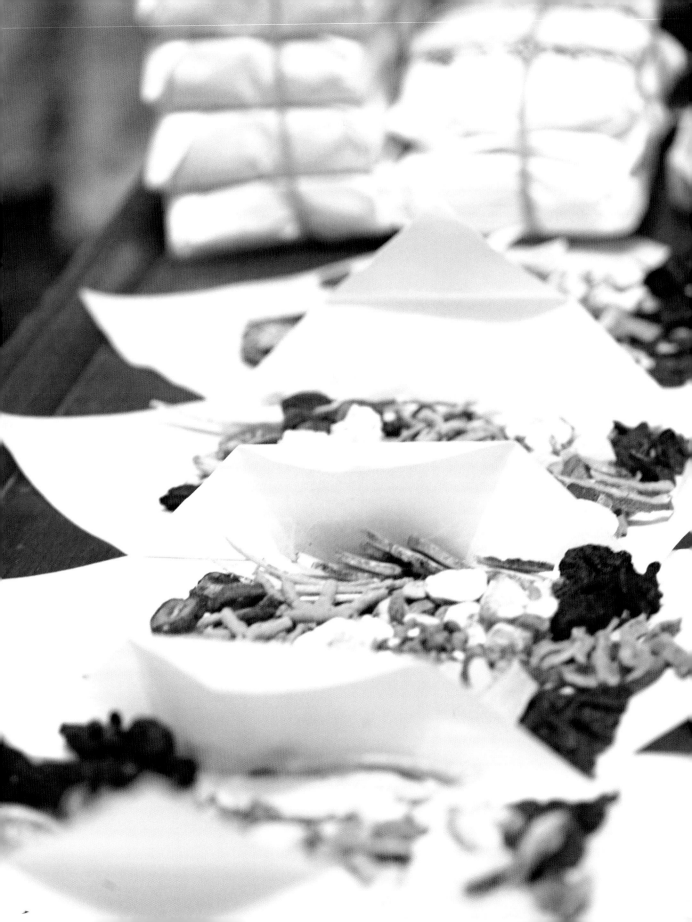

A Way of Life
Traditional Chinese Medicine in Malaysia

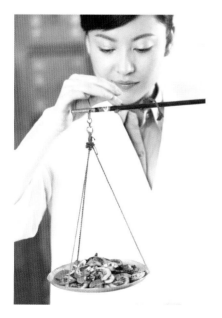

Opposite Traditional Chinese medicine has long had a place in Malaysian culture.

Below Plants and herbs are processed and prepared in several ways in traditional Chinese medicine. The dosage of herbs is usually adjusted to each patient, depending on age, gender and other factors.

Although traditional Chinese medicine (TCM) is only now becoming well known and understood globally, it has long had a place in the culture of the Chinese (and to a certain extent other populations) in Malaysia. TCM manifests itself in many different ways: in the cooking of particular recipes at home; in a visit to one of the country's numerous reflexology centers or *sinseh* shops in its shopping malls; or in the hundreds of aromatic, sometimes musty-smelling, Chinese apothecaries where staff weigh up little packets of exotic roots and powders and transfer them in brown paper envelopes to busy shoppers.

Such scenes are commonplace all over the country. Reflexology is seen by many Asians as one of the best ways to sustain the long-term health of internal organs as well as a quick pick-me-up. Similarly, cooking up a traditional tonic for vitality such as chicken soup with astragalus, red dates and wolfberries is commonplace in Chinese households when one wants a quick health boost. Preparing a mixture of crushed pearl and vitamin E oil and using it as a complexion brightener is another weekly ritual for many—after all, people say, if Cixi, the last Empress Dowager of China, used pure freshwater pearl dust to maintain smooth flawless skin, why shouldn't we?

So how did these Chinese practices come to be part and parcel of everyday life in Malaysia? How did they get there?

An Admiral's Bounty

In 1409, admiral Zheng He's third voyage to the Indian Ocean was partly inspired by the need to collect medicinal products that were in short supply at that time in China. The Ming Dynasty was experiencing a growing population, poor public health conditions and shocking outbreaks of infectious diseases, especially measles and smallpox. Millions were dying in rampant epidemics.

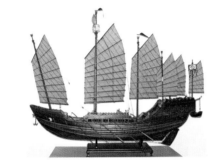

Above Model of a treasure ship in Zheng He's fleet.
Right Statue of Zheng He in Nanjing, China.

On this trip, Zheng He's fleet of enormous treasure ships traveled with 180 medical specialists—from physicians to herb collectors and herbal processing experts. A 17th-century historian, Zhang Xie, covered this voyage in *Dongxi Yangkao* (Study of Eastern and Western Oceans) and noted that the natural medicines collected from Indonesia, Borneo and the Malay Peninsula included camphor, frankincense, myrrh, musk, sandalwood, pepper, ginger, sulfur, aloeswood (*gaharu*), rhinoceros horn, deer antler, birds' nest, clove, cinnamon, cardamom, patchouli, storax gum and benzoin. Kelantan's aloeswood and Sarawak's birds' nests from the Niah caves were renowned for their high quality. These products were processed on board, so they were ready for immediate medicinal use upon arrival in China.

Trade and Migration: Spreading the Word

It's known that active trade was occurring between India and China since at least the beginning of the 1st century CE. Because the Malay Peninsula lies strategically between these two nations, it was a natural stop-off point during sea voyages. Archeological evidence and historical data show that the Chinese thought of the Malay Peninsula as a region rich with natural exotica: gold, pearls, rhinoceros horns, tortoise shells, spices and fragrant woods were only some of its sought-after treasures.

At some point, although scholars are not exactly sure when, an informal type of tribute system began: silks and porcelain were exchanged for goods from the Malay Peninsula, and by the 5th century, Malay diplomatic envoys were being welcomed into China to further the ties. The various Chinese *materia medica* already printed at this time list many Southeast Asian rainforest products as having medicinal value, but it is not known whether Chinese traders were motivated by the medicinal values of these items or whether they were sought after for other reasons. Fragrant ingredients such as cinnamon and nutmeg were used as culinary spices and for incense, but they were also added to herbal formulations for therapy.

What is known, however, is that Buddhist Chinese monks traveling to India to further their religious studies routinely broke their sea voyages in Southeast Asia and collected items specifically for their therapeutic benefits. Of noted importance were the activities of the monks Faxian (5th century) and Yiqing (7th century), who very likely stayed in the coastal areas of Kedah, Terengganu and Kelantan. Their diaries describe Kadaram as a place of great felicity, civilization and abundance. And from the 7th century onwards, tributary gifts and trading for natural exotica were inspired to a large degree by the therapeutic properties that these items were believed to confer.

Buddhism played a large part in these therapeutic quests, and many collected items were stored in major Buddhist monasteries. Tang Dynasty records indicate that the Malay Peninsula and Borneo had the best medicinal quality sandalwood, betel nut, storax gum, guggul resin, camphor, musk and patchouli. As noted in the 10th-century *Kaibao Bencao* (*materia medica* of the Kai Bao era), a handful of these natural medicines were given names with the prefix dragon that remain until this day. It was believed that these precious items were gifts from the lively dragons of the Southern Seas, so, camphor is known as 'dragon's brain', ambergris as 'dragon's spittle' and rattan gum as 'dragon's blood', among others.

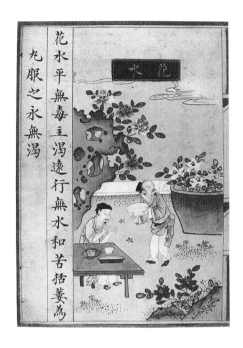

Above Illustration of 'flower water', a dietetic herbal, from *Shiwu Bencao* (*materia dietetica*), dating from the Ming period (1368–1644).

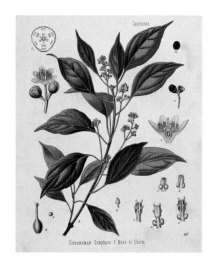

The most popular of these traded items were the aromatics used by Buddhist and Daoist monks. For example, camphor and musk incense was burned to wake up dull senses and enhance deep meditation, and also as an offering during prayer, for spiritual purification or just to dispel foul odors. From the Chinese medical perspective, such aromatics were also ingested to dispel dampness and phlegm. Due to the sedentary lifestyle of monastic living and prolonged meditation, there's a tendency for excessive dampness to accumulate in the body, which, with time, disrupts proper digestion and gives rise to all kinds of stagnation. TCM advocates that most aromatics attend to this specific health imbalance, resulting in a renewed lightness in the body.

Of course, with time, some of these travelers turned into settlers. The earliest record of a significant Chinese settlement in Malaya came in the early 1400s when a small trading community was founded in Melaka. Strategically located between the Spice Islands of Indonesia and India, Melaka was

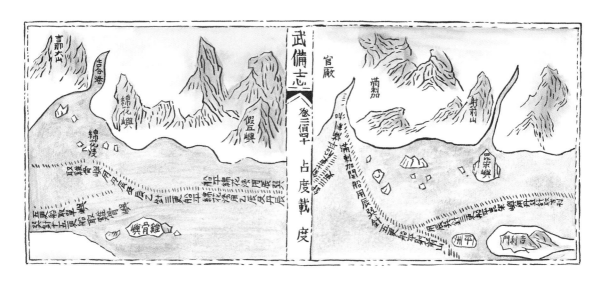

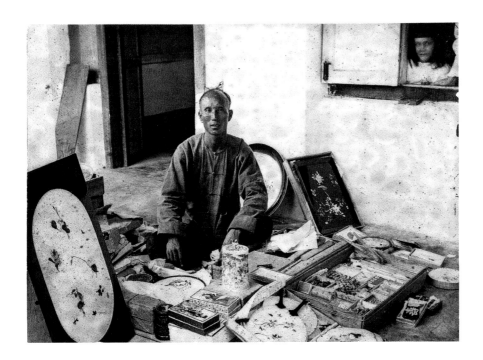

the busiest entrepôt for the thriving Chinese maritime trade at that time. Ming dynasty diplomatic ties with the Melaka ruler, mediated by the maritime admiral Zheng He in 1409, also enhanced the image of Melaka as an exalted kingdom in its own right.

As its importance grew, so did Melaka's population, with more and more Chinese traders moving in. Warehouses and granaries were built to house goods bought in Southeast Asia and India, which were later transferred on to China. The Chinese who remained in Melaka married local native women and their progeny became the first generation of Peranakan (local Straits-born) Chinese in the Malay Peninsula. In the ensuing centuries, this community prospered and became highly influential; they developed an extremely elaborate social, medicinal and culinary culture that continues to this day.

Opposite, above Botanical drawing of the camphor plant.

Opposite, below Sailing paths in and out of the Melaka estuary and sailing directions, depicted in this chart from the Chinese military compendium, *Wu Pei Chih* ('Notes on Military Preparedness'), which dates from the first half of the 15th century. The name Melaka is inscribed above a representation of the hill (later known as Saint Paul's Hill) overlooking the harbor.

Above Chinese street hawker in Taiping, Perak, in 1886.

During the 19th to the early 20th century, China's last dynasty, the chaotic Qing, wrought untold misery on the Chinese population. Many people fled the country, some paying their way out of China and others leaving as contract laborers. At the same time, new economic opportunities in colonial British Malaya created employment for these waves of southern Chinese mass migrations that continued up until the early 20th century. As a result, large congregations of Chinese settled in the urban areas of Penang, Perak, Selangor and Johor.

Being away from their native country, these expatriate populations formed close-knit communities through associations, clans and support groups. Naturally, their own cultural, medicinal, religious and other practices gave succor; in sickness and in health, they turned to what they knew to sustain them.

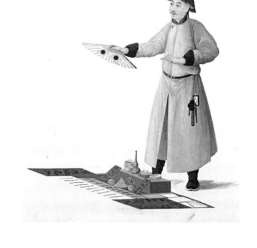

What is TCM?

Even though history shows how certain Chinese traditional practices came to the Malay Peninsula and survive today, it's important to explain a little about the history, philosophy and development of TCM in China. This throws light on the various TCM practices that flourish in today's Malaysia. It is especially relevant in light of the fact that a modern version of TCM is gaining serious legitimacy worldwide.

Firstly, it needs to be noted that TCM did not develop homogenously; rather, scholars, philosophers, monks, emperors, alchemists, naturalists, politicians and others all contributed to its body of accumulated knowledge. Secondly, even though it is generally noted as having a 5,000-year-old

Above An image of a Chinese medicine seller taken from a volume of Chinese drawings, c. 1800.

Opposite, above A Chinese good luck talisman with the *yin-yang* symbol and the eight trigrams (*ba gua*).

Opposite, below A meridian map detailing the acupoints and the circulation of *qi* in the body.

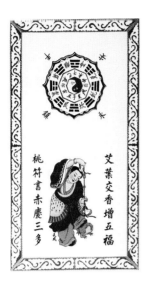

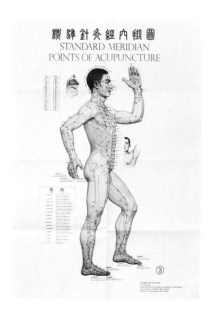

STANDARD MERIDIAN
POINTS OF ACUPUNCTURE

documented history, the clearest archeological evidence of TCM actually dates from the Shang Dynasty about 3,500 years ago. From this period, tens of thousands of turtle shells and cattle bones inscribed with information relating to treatments for health complaints—problematic eyes, headache, toothache and the like—have been found. These are the first definitive TCM 'texts'.

Over the ensuing centuries, these early texts were followed by various medical listings, philosophical treatises and divinatory texts that attempted to explain spiritual, evolutionary and medicinal matters. In essence, they were all trying to make sense of the world. It would be too cumbersome to list these, but suffice it to say that, through this vast body of thinking, a number of underlying concepts came to be accepted as fact: the concept of two opposing forces of *yin* and *yang*; the desire for longevity; the idea of *qi* or a vital life force that flows along a network of channels within the body; the thought that medicine should be preventative rather than curative; and the importance of diet and herbalism, among others.

Over the centuries, these varying ideas loosely took hold, with empirical evidence and research continuously adding to the body of knowledge about the human body and its relation to the world and universe. Various therapies were developed to facilitate human health and, by the Tang Dynasty (618–907), a highly sophisticated Chinese medical system existed. In fact, China was considered the medical center of Asia. Its consolidation into a homogenously packaged TCM system with standardized terminology for diagnosis and treatment did not occur, however, until well into the 20th century.

Purifying the Air, Chinese Style

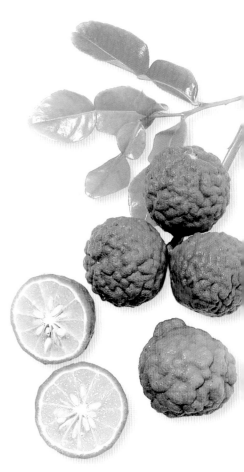

As the Chinese settled in the Malay Peninsula through various waves of migration, they began to experiment with local plants for a variety of uses—culinary, medicinal and environmental. In today's Malaysia, local Chinese generally use fresh herbs for non-chronic problems such as nose bleeds and minor cuts, wounds and insect bites. Long-term health issues are very likely attended to with imported TCM herbs that are widely available in *sinseh* shops.

In the field of purifying their immediate environment, the Chinese found plenty of local plants on hand. As the air and climate in the tropics were very different from their home environment, they felt the need to create an atmosphere conducive to both mental and physical health. Thus, purifying the air in the home in order to eliminate odors, enhance mental clarity, promote sleep and generally create a cleaner atmosphere was a priority.

So, which local plants were useful to them? How did they go about their aims?

Jerangau (*Acorus calamus, left*) is considered a warm, sensory-opening herb in TCM; the roots are often soaked in rice wine with ginger to create a tonic that improves sleep and clears the brain. It was also used, along with *selasih* leaves (*Ocimum basilicum*), in ritual smoking to purify the environment. Even today, the whole jerangau plant, along with whole green onion stalks, is hung on Chinese doorframes during the summer solstice in June to purify the air and get rid of insects. Interestingly, selasih is added to burning charcoal by Taoist healers during ritual smoking to purify a person who complains of chest tightness and constriction of the heart.

Another environmental purifier is Kaffir lime or *limau purut* (*Citrus hystrix, above right*). Today, it is proven that essential oil obtained from the fresh peel of Kaffir lime when permeating the atmosphere leads to increased alertness and activity. Indeed, in Japan, it is often placed in air-conditioning ducts in factories to promote productivity! In Chinese

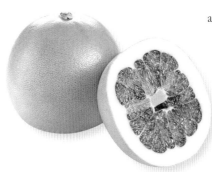

households in Malaysia, the zest of Kaffir lime was added to bath water with the petals of five colored flowers as a cleansing agent for those who had attended either a funeral or a birth. The fresh, tangy scent permeated the atmosphere too.

Another local citrus fruit known as an environmental cleanser was a type of giant grapefruit known as a pomelo (*Citrus grandis, left*). Dried peel of the pomelo was used for purificatory smoking of both the house and its residents. The fresh leaf, similar to that of the auspicious gourd *hu lu* was, and still is, used as an offering.

TCM Adaptations in Malaysian Society

Although Malaysia's 'official' medicine is Western, the traditional healing practices of Malays, Chinese, Indians and other indigenous groups have been used as a primary and, at times, complementary healthcare system for centuries. As a result, the practice of self-care healing within the home is a major part of the cultural fabric of Malaysia.

As the Chinese comprise the country's second largest ethnic group (in 2007, about 25 percent of Malaysia's population was Chinese), it is not surprising that their traditional approaches to healthcare survive and flourish. Chinese healing practices are seen primarily in three areas—everyday life, trading and charitable organizations.

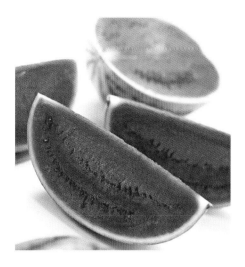

Above Watermelon is considered a 'cooling' food by the Chinese, and is thus useful in hot weather.

TCM in Everyday Life

The daily life of Malaysian Chinese society has been prominently influenced by Chinese medicine in two particular spheres: the culinary arts and trauma-care techniques. In TCM, all foods are deemed medicinal, so most Chinese know about the therapeutic properties of common foods at least to a certain extent. The 'hot–cold' nature of foods is most familiar to the average Chinese, while some of the more well informed can further determine if a particular food item will increase or decrease 'wind', improve dryness or increase dampness.

Take watermelon, for instance. Many Chinese are familiar with the idea that watermelon is a 'cold'-nature fruit, useful during hot weather. Some may also know that it is considered moisturizing and influences the lungs and stomach. As such, not only is watermelon useful during hot weather, it is also suitable if a person has a dry cough and a sore throat. It is also eaten to lessen the burning sensation experienced after a particularly hot and spicy meal.

Another common spice, fresh ginger, is widely used in the kitchen and not just for its flavor. When two to three slices are added to stir-fried bean sprouts, ginger tones down the 'cold' nature of bean sprouts. Added to seafood, ginger will prevent seafood poisoning. After menstruation, girls are given a nourishing soup made from Chinese angelica, ginger and chicken to replenish the blood.

Herbal teas, mostly cooling in nature and made palatable with the addition of rock sugar, are drunk liberally to counteract the heat and humidity of Malaysia. For instance, sweet momordica fruit with prunella spikes is regularly boiled to cleanse the system; chrysanthemum with wolfberries is taken to nourish the eyes; and a licorice and honeysuckle flower decoction is thought to quell a fever in its initial stages. Much of this type of information is orally handed down from mother to daughter, from the elders to the younger generations—and is innovatively incorporated into everyday meals.

Below In addition to adding flavor, fresh ginger balances the 'cold' nature of certain foods.

Bottom Herbal soups are commonly consumed by Chinese to nourish and replenish the blood.

Opposite Herbal teas are mostly 'cooling' in nature and should be taken frequently to counteract heat.

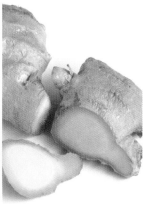

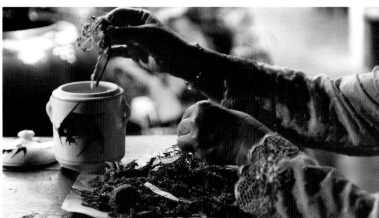

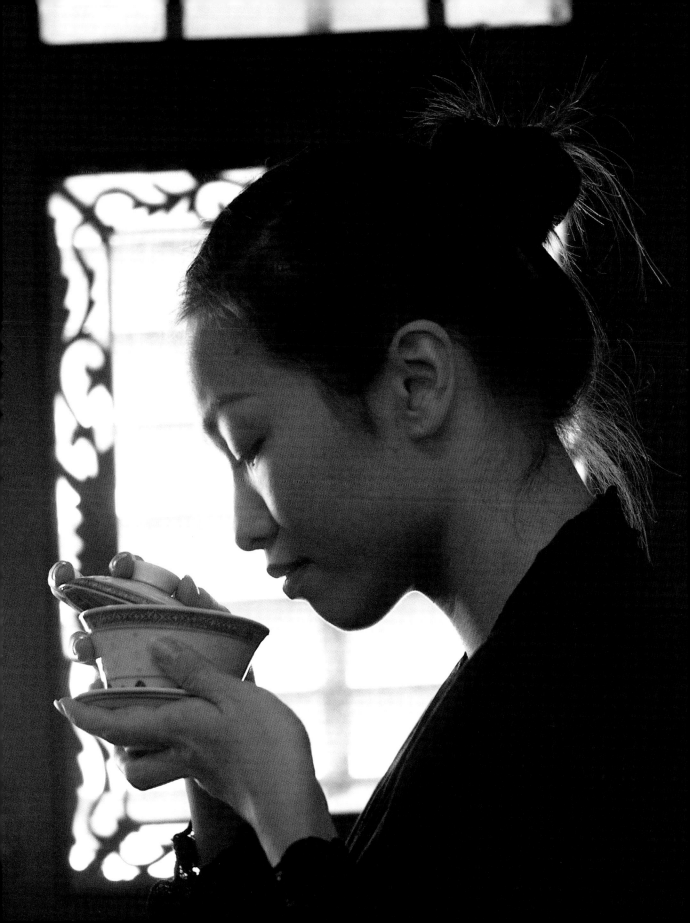

Martial Arts' Injuries: Local Herbs to Dull the Pain

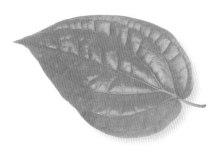

Local herbs proved invaluable to the newly settled Chinese migrants when they suffered from sprains, breaks, fractures and the attendant aches and pains resulting from martial arts injuries. Some herbs were harvested fresh, while others were obtained dried and prepared in many of the burgeoning *sinseh* shops. If the local herbal apothecary could cut out the time-consuming digging, washing, cleaning, drying and preparing of plants and sell them at a reasonable price, so much the better.

Today, the tradition continues with local plants often favored over chemical substitutes. After all, they represent centuries of healing traditions, and should not be underestimated.

Using the whole dried plant including the flower, *bunga susung* (*Ervatamia divaricata*) is helpful in the final stages of trauma care treatment, especially if fractures are involved. Boiled with some other nourishing herbs, it is used to reduce pain, excess heat and swelling. Another herb helpful at such a time, especially if there is pain in the lower back, is *pokok tunjuk langit* (*Helminthosachys zeylanica*). Called the 'centipede plant' as the flower when faded looks like a centipede on the floor, it is made into a decoction for such patients.

If the injuries are more superficial in the form of bruises and swelling, *cili padi* (*Capsicum frutescens, below left*) are taken from the garden and put to good use. The plant's leaves are pounded and dry fried in a wok with a crushed chili and a few grams of *da huang* or dried Chinese rhubarb root. Once a paste forms, it is placed directly on the painful area while still warm to act as an anti-inflammatory and pain reliever.

Also useful as an external application for sprains is the fruit of *kaca piring* (*Gardenia augusta, below right*). Mashed up and added to a whisked egg white, it alleviates pain and reduces swelling. Another anti-inflammatory is the dried mushroom known as *kulat kayu* (*Ganoderma lucidum*). Research shows it to be a potent anti-cancer agent and its Latin name signifies its value in providing a healthy and radiant (*ludicum*) skin (*ganoderma*).

In Malaysian Chinese communities, it is used in TCM formulations for all forms of aches and pains especially for weakness and frailty or when a person is recuperating from a long illness. But martial arts practitioners find it helpful too. Steeped in hot water with red dates, it is drunk as a tea throughout the day.

Of course, the ubiquitous *Piper betle* or *sirih (above)*, considered a warm *qi* activator, shouldn't be overlooked. It is used both internally and externally to remove 'wind' and reduce pain. Internally, the dried leaves and stems are boiled with fresh ginger to produce a tea, while the fresh or dried leaves and stems are cooked with sesame oil and other herbs like citronella to make an ointment for external application. In martial arts circles, sirih liniment is considered an essential.

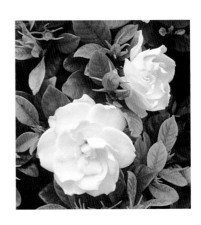

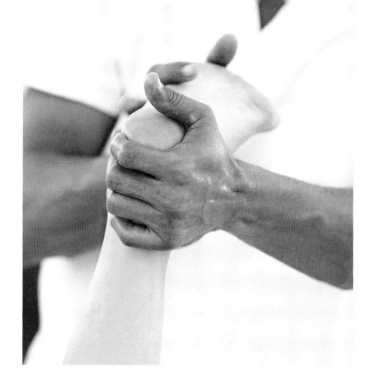

If such herbal dietary healthcare is considered the domain of womenfolk, Chinese medicinal trauma-care is reserved for men. Especially prominent in the vibrant Chinese martial art sub-culture, it has its roots in the early migrant communities' self-defense practices. Martial art practitioners, especially masters, were well versed in what is known as *dieda* or 'hit-and-fall medicine'.

Injuries acquired during martial arts practice and competitions, as well as from non-related events like occupational accidents, are often treated by martial art masters. Although treatments for bruises, dislocations and fractures are the primary area of expertise, masters also have specialized knowledge of Chinese herbs and of acu-points and vulnerable areas of the body. The throat, epigastrium (upper middle region of the abdomen) and armpits, for example, can be deadly when hit or injured; cupping, massage or herbal applications are often prescribed in such cases, with splints and traction also used to align structural imbalances.

The underlying principle of hit-and-fall medicine is to restore *qi* flow to relieve obstruction that, in turn, causes stagnation.

Above Injuries sustained during martial arts practice and occupational accidents are often treated by martial art masters.

Below A watercolor depicting a patient receiving manipulative treatment for a pain in the shoulder.

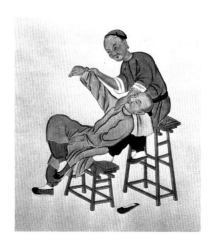

A Bright Red Resin: Dragon's Blood

The name 'dragon's blood' may sound like an ingredient in a witch's brew or magic potion, and an aura of mystery prevailed around the trade of these bright red plant resins: different plants from distant places in the world have been known as the source of this precious panacea.

Dragon's blood is mentioned in various ancient texts for its medicinal value, and it has been used in cultures as far apart as Rome and China. In the 1st-century work, *Periplus of the Erythraean Sea*, dragon's blood was mentioned as a product of the Yemeni island of Socotra in the Indian Ocean. Indeed, Socotra (also known as the Island of Dragon's Blood) provides a source from its indigenous tree *Drecaena cinnabari*.

Dragon's blood in Southeast Asia and in China has been used as a general cure-all, employed for healing wounds.

However, dragon's blood has also long been traded out of Malay ports, and here it is derived from the immature fruit of rattan palms in the genus *Daemonorops*. This palm flourishes throughout the Malay Archipelago where it is known as *jerang*.

Therefore, it is likely that ancient Rome sourced its dragon's blood from Socotra, but Han China and subsequent Chinese dynasties are thought to have obtained their supply from the Malay world.

In Malaysia, until today, dragon's blood resin is obtained by picking the cherry-sized, unripe fruits, which carry a protective layer of bright red resin. The dried fruits are placed in bags and then beaten to dislodge the resin. The resinous powder thus obtained is sifted and warmed so that it can be molded into sticks or rolled into solid balls before being sold.

Dragon's blood in Southeast Asia and in China—made from the resin sourced from Malaysia's *Daemonorops* species—has been used as a general cure-all, a wound healer, to lower fever, and to cure such ailments as diarrhea, dysentery and stomach ulcers.

Current research indicates that dragon's blood from the *Daemonorops* genus has anti-coagulant properties, thus confirming the medicinal value attributed to it in former times.

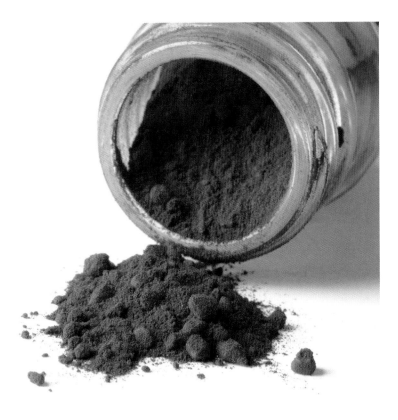

Left Dragon's blood powder.

Herbs used in this area also require special expertise. For instance, injuries below the waist are treated with a formula that contains arcyranthes root; injuries above the diaphragm need safflower and bupleurum; for the abdomen, rhubarb and peach kernels are useful; and for the back along the spine, notopterygium root is compulsory. Post-injury care, after pain has subsided, is equally important: TCM advocates that it is imperative to restore optimal functioning of the liver at this point. If the liver is not balanced, it's believed that the whole musculature will be weak, thus inviting further injuries, sprains and falls.

Such specialists have served the Malaysian community well for decades as they provide low cost orthopedic care for simple accidents and, more importantly, serve as first-aid providers in rural areas where hospitals are scarce or inaccessible.

Another unique example of a Malaysian adaptation of Chinese health practices is seen in Peranakan Chinese society. This once prominent community, found mainly in Melaka and Penang, employs a self-care approach to health that was influenced by both the Malays and the migrant Chinese that they generally employed as cooks or maids. Over time, a unique blend of Malay and Chinese practices developed— and continues to this day.

Beauty techniques and post-natal care were especially prominent in Peranakan culture as most Peranakan women (known as Nyonyas) were homemakers. For example, a post-natal foot massage with oil is of Malay influence, while the drinking of herbal tea consisting of red dates, black beans and codonopsis root (*Codonopsis pilosula*) came from the Chinese tradition. Floral and lime showers to cleanse the post-natal mother originated from Malay tradition, while the celebratory

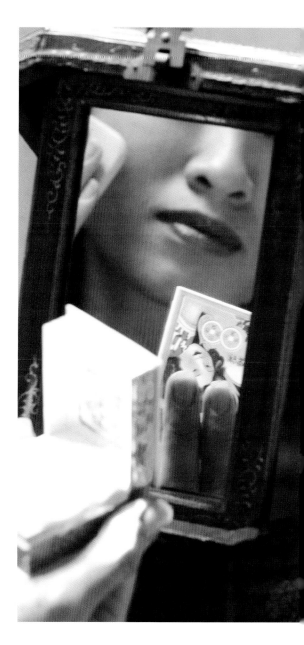

Above Peranakan women are renowned for their beauty care techniques, among other things.

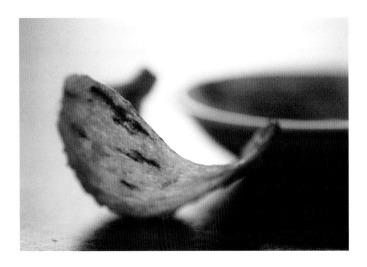

announcement of the full moon baby at the ancestral altar is of Chinese influence.

In the early 20th century, when the Peranakans reached their apogee of social and economic standing, they had a penchant for premium Chinese medicines. Nyonyas would grind tiny white pearls into powder, add them to rice powder and apply them on the face. They would regularly consume edible birds' nests, a rare and expensive commodity, as a complexion booster. Steaming slices of (imported) American ginseng was also common in Peranakan households; the men, called Babas, were encouraged to drink such ginseng decoctions, as they needed extra vitality due to their heavy work schedules.

Such exotic (and expensive) natural therapeutics have withstood the test of time. The scientific benefits have now been established and the formulae refined. After all, what could be more beguiling than applying natural pearl powders renowned for their rejuvenating and healing properties with scented essential oils to cool and refine the skin?

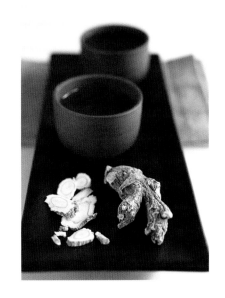

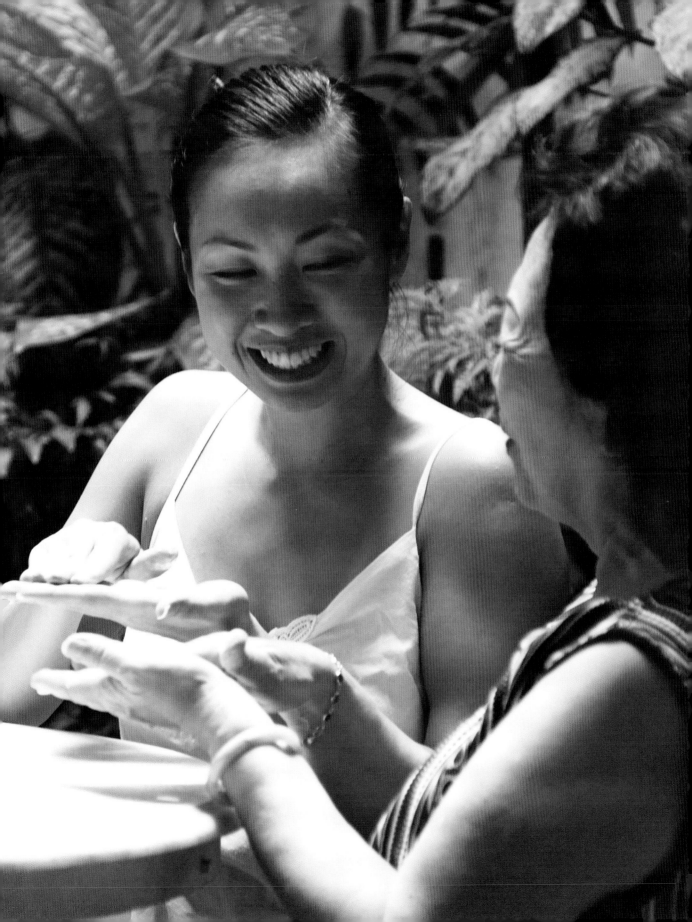

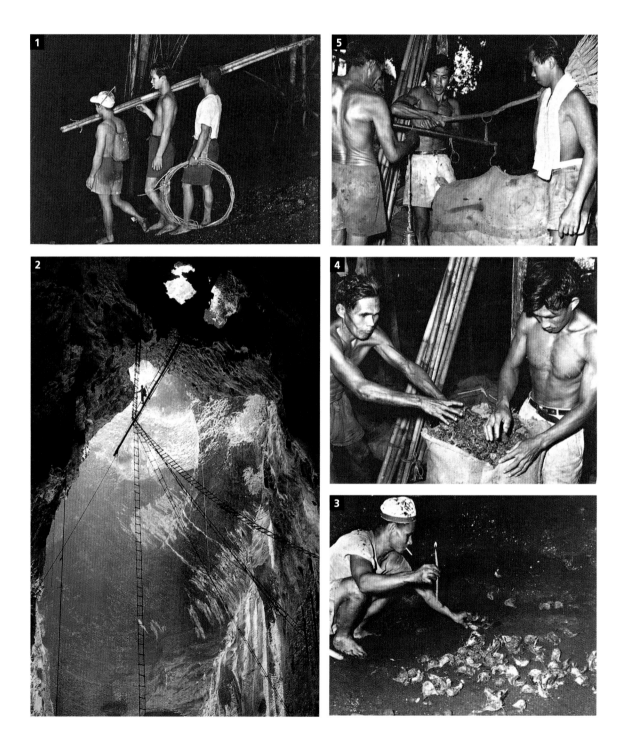

Swiftlets and Birds' Nest Soup

A luxury ingredient reserved for special occasions in Chinese households is birds' nest soup, a clear consommé. Containing nests composed of the dried spittle of cave-dwelling swiftlets, the attraction of the dish is in its remedial and restorative tonic value, the knowledge that it is a rare and expensive commodity and the fact that it was served as a delicacy in the Imperial Court of China for countless centuries.

Included as gifts of tribute from Malay rulers to the Chinese Emperor, along with precious hardwoods and rare medicinal herbs, the most commonly harvested nests are those of the white-nest swiftlet (*Aerodramus fuciphagus*) and the black-nest swiftlet (*Aerodramus maximus*). Both the white nests and the rarer 'red blood' nests are believed to be rich in nutrients traditionally considered to provide health benefits. Taken to aid digestion, as an aphrodisiac, to alleviate asthma, sharpen mental focus and provide overall benefit to the human immune system, the nests are finding their way into skincare regimes as well.

Swiftlet nests are traditionally harvested from Malaysian caves, principally the enormous limestone caves at Gomantong in Sabah and at Niah in Sarawak, as well as from caves in Indonesia and southern Thailand. Their collection is a precarious business, with workers risking life and limb climbing up shaky rattan ladders dangling from the ceiling of caves and inching along bamboo ladders to gather the nests. As many are some 60 meters (200 feet) high, the risks are considerable.

The nests are built during the breeding season by the male swiftlet over a period of about five weeks. They take the shape of a shallow cup stuck to the cave wall. Composed of interwoven strands of salivary cement, the nests of both species contain high levels of calcium, iron, potassium and magnesium.

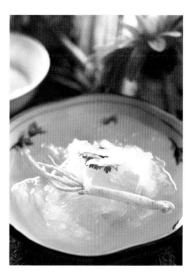

Hong Kong and the United States are the largest importers of swiftlet nests. In Hong Kong, a bowl of birds' nest soup can cost between US$30 and US$100. A kilogram of the more common white nest can cost up to US$2,000, while a kilo of the rarer red blood nest can cost up to US$10,000. The white nests are commonly treated with a red pigment, but buyers have developed sophisticated methods to identify such adulterated nests.

With increasing worldwide demand, traditional cave sources have been supplanted by purpose-built concrete nesting houses. Normally constructed in urban areas near the sea since the birds are inclined to flock in such places, they are easily accessible. Swiftlet nest farming has developed into a major industry mainly in Malaysia and nearby Indonesia, and the nests are usually exported to Hong Kong, now the center of the world trade.

Opposite Rattan ladders are erected to reach the nests (1–2). The collected nests are then cleaned, weighed and packed for export (3–5).

Above Birds' nest can be prepared in many ways, but it is most commonly cooked as a sweet, soup-based dessert.

Right Birds' nests can fetch high prices due to their rarity and nutrients.

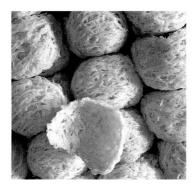

Malaysia has a rich repository of Chinese medicinal plants, such as betel nut, camphor wood and cardamom, which were at one time highly sought after by Imperial China.

Trade and Charity: The spread of TCM

Luckily, Malaysia has proved a rich repository of Chinese medicinal plants: betel nut, camphor wood, cardamom, cinnamon, cloves, nutmeg, patchouli, pepper and red sandalwood are all native to Malaysia, and, as noted, they were at one time highly sought after by Imperial China. Other more common herbs used in Chinese healthcare like hibiscus, calamus, lemongrass, turmeric, aloe vera, galangal and citronella are easily grown in back yards and harvested fresh as and when needed. Even herbs like ginseng, licorice and astragalus, as well as time-tested patent medicines, are widely available in Malaysia, as trade brought these items from China.

There are currently at least 1,000 stores in Malaysia that are involved in the trade of traditional Chinese medicinal products. Operated primarily by Cantonese and Hakka groups, they have served an important and practical role in Malaysian society in general, and to the Chinese in particular. The widespread presence of retail outlets along with the direct marketing business that sells Chinese medicinal products nationwide have encouraged those outside the Chinese community to further explore the use of TCM. Also keeping TCM very much alive and kicking are the Chinese practitioners and dealers associations in Malaysia which run degree-granting programs in TCM in conjunction with Chinese universities, thus producing a whole cadre of Malaysian Chinese TCM doctors.

Furthermore, the Buddhist ideals of charity and merit making, that have influenced classical Chinese medical think-ing since the introduction of Buddhism to China 2,000 years ago, continue to this day. Practitioners of the healing arts were encouraged to help others without charge, both to gain merit

Opposite There are currently at least 1,000 stores in Malaysia that are involved in the trade of traditional Chinese medicinal products.

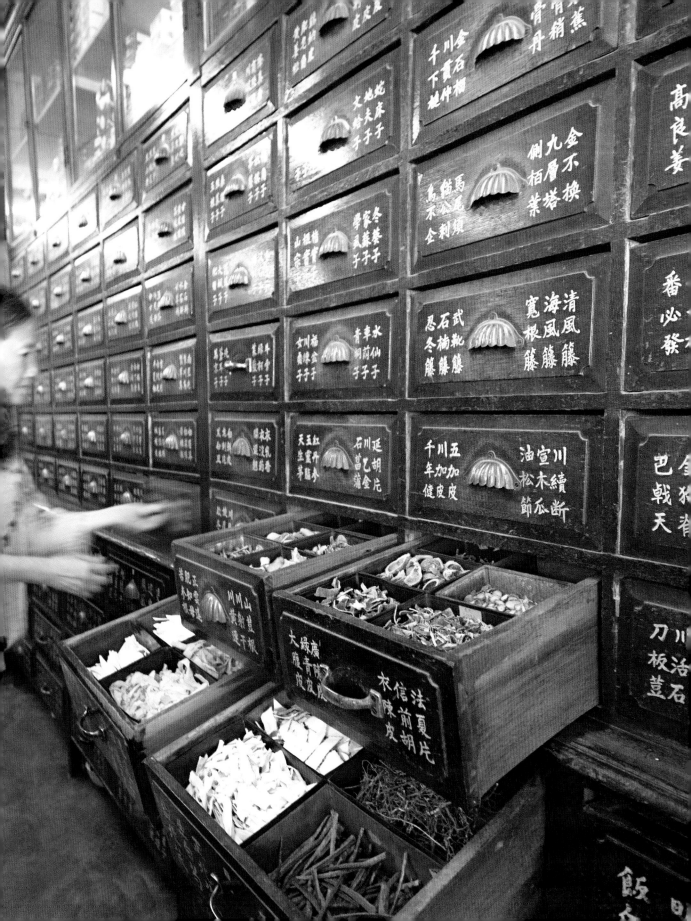

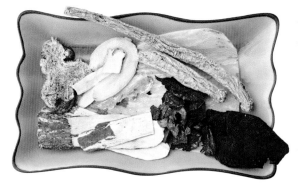

The general public is aware that Chinese medicine has a place in their lives because, inevitably, family members or close friends have benefited from the practice, either from services rendered professionally, freely or in a self-care manner.

for themselves and relieve the sickness of those less fortunate than themselves. This tradition continues to this day. There are charitable Chinese medical institutions, set up decades ago in Kuala Lumpur and Penang, that serve the poor irrespective of race and religion. Many well-financed temples in Malaysia also provide free TCM clinics where volunteers donate their skill and time to treat patients without charge.

The Future

It's clear that Chinese medicinal practices will continue to flourish and grow in Malaysia, especially since TCM is fast gaining wider global credibility and people are becoming more aware of its therapeutic benefits.

In a local context, TCM has been serving the health needs of Malaysia's population for centuries. The general public is very much aware that Chinese medicine has a place in their lives, because, inevitably, family members or close friends have benefited from the practice, either from services rendered professionally, freely or in a self-care manner. And most are aware that TCM acts as a complement with or an alternative to Western allopathic care—and doesn't replace it completely.

In addition, the Peranakan experience has added another dimension. The rich fusion of Malay and Chinese traditions that gave birth to the fascinating Peranakan culture throws light on the ongoing process of evolution in healthcare traditions. Expect to see more and more Malaysian dimensions of TCM in the future: as practices become further adapted to local conditions and medicinal materials, more exotic, exciting rituals are sure to emerge.

Sinseh Shops: Serving the Community

Sinseh shops, found across the length and breadth of Malaysia, are stores that sell traditional Chinese medicinal products. Derived from the Hokkien variant of the Mandarin term *xian sheng*, sinseh is a traditional term of respect for a learned person, doctor or professor.

Originally set up to import and sell key TCM products and ingredients unavailable in Malaysia, sinseh shops are not herbal apothecaries in the real sense of the word. Rather, they're a combination of the Chinese grocer and herbal healthcare retailer. Operated primarily by Malaysians of Chinese descent, it is estimated that there are at least 1,000 sinseh stores in Malaysia, where they have a distinct appeal for customers of Malay and Indian ethnic origin as well as for ethnic Chinese.

Early Chinese migrants to Malaysia were able to practice their natural system of healthcare simply because the necessary products and services were readily available.

Many herbs used in traditional Chinese medicine are native plants of Malaysia, while other plants are grown locally. Sinseh shops sell all these, along with plenty of Chinese imports. A fine example of a sinseh shop made good is the case of the oldest existing company in Malaysia involved in the trade of traditional Chinese medicines. Founded by a Cantonese, who migrated from Guangdong in China to Malaya in the 1870s, the gentleman in question established himself firstly as a tin miner, then founded a grocery in Gopeng in the state of Perak. To help his sickly workers who were primarily opium smokers, he incorporated a Chinese medicine section, and started bringing in herbs and patent medicines from China. Over the years, the company developed into a fully-fledged, premium grade Chinese herbal apothecary and is now a public-listed company in Singapore, with a total of 120 outlets in Malaysia, Singapore and Hong Kong.

Other sinseh shops have less lofty ambitions: many are owner-operated small concerns that continue to serve people in their immediate locality. Some are affiliated with TCM doctors who may have an adjacent consultation room.

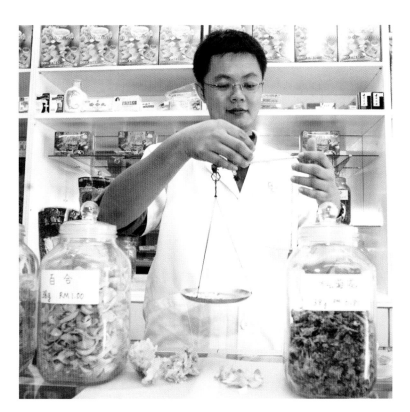

Left Originally set up to import and sell key TCM products and ingredients unavailable in Malaysia, *sinseh* shops are a combination of the Chinese grocer and herbal healthcare retailer.

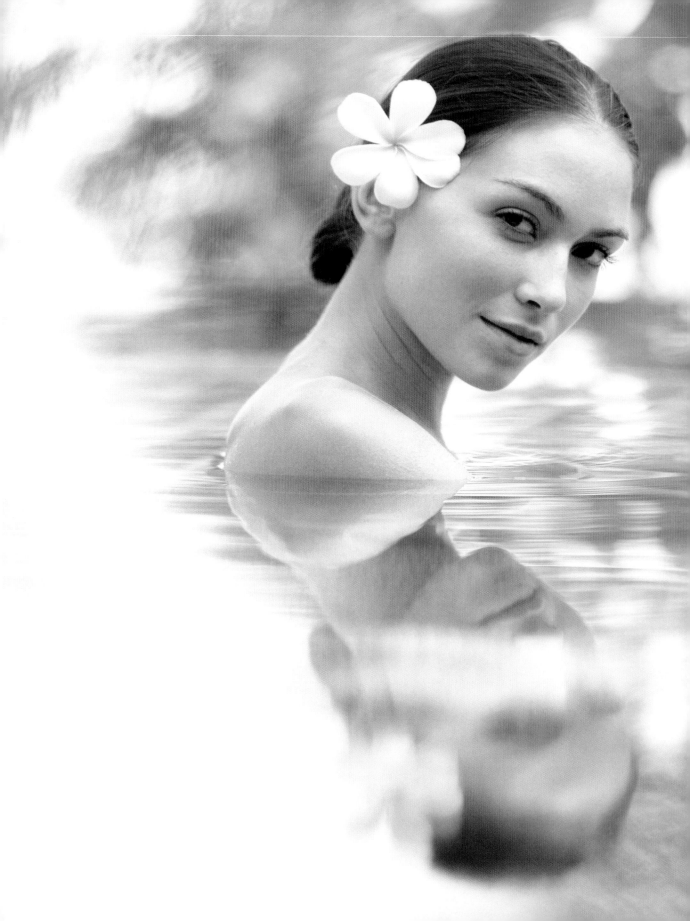

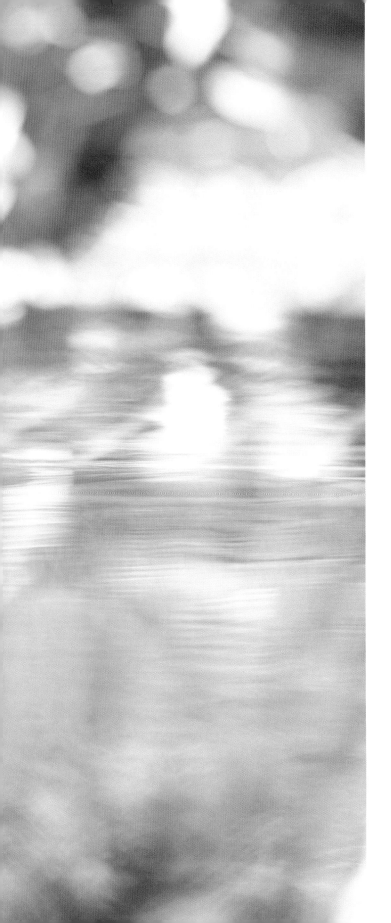

The Spa in Malaysia

Returning the body to equilibrium—
through time-honored rituals and age-
old botanical remedies—is the focus
of the spa in Malaysia. Drawing on
the country's holistic medical systems,
in the form of Malay healthcare,
Ayurveda and traditional Chinese
medicine, treatments are a mix of the
therapeutic, the rejuvenating and the
relaxing. Whether it's a meditative
massage, a session of a Malay martial
art, a fabulous floral bath or an exotic
facial, the experience soothes the heart
and uplifts the mind. For complete
immersion in the country's ancient
healing philosophy, there is no better
place than the spa.

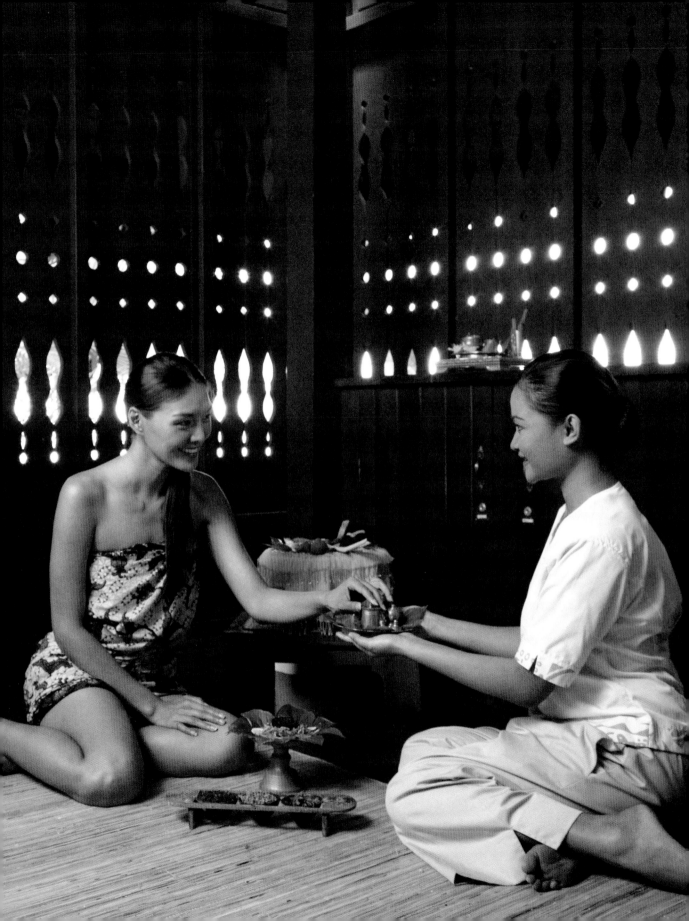

Havens of Healing
The Spa and Spa Treatments in Malaysia Today

The experience of lying on soft *batik* in an open-sided pavilion receiving care and caresses from both a traditional Malay massage and cooling breezes coming directly off the nearby ocean isn't something from a fantasy film. In a Malay spa, it can be a reality. The combination of healing hands, age-old formulae and a beautifully designed tropical environment has the ability to lure clients into an other-worldly state.

Certainly, it seems a dream-like state—a highly pleasurable one—but it is, in fact, entirely tangible. The mystic masseur has the ability to weave magic; his or her touch grounds the experience fully in the present, suspending time as it were. Circulation speeds up, the muscles are toned and stretched, the scents of spicy oils calm and soothe, and the mind and body become one.

The benefits of such an experience—physically, mentally, and emotionally—cannot be underestimated. Alternately relaxing and stimulating, it is, however, no miracle wonder trick. Rather, it takes its cue from centuries of tradition.

The Malaysian Spa Experience

Such is the state of the Malaysian spa today. On the one hand, it's a modern source of wellness, offering holistic healing

Previous pages The spa allows one to return the body and mind to a state of equilibrium.

Opposite A spa therapist discusses the efficacy of traditional Malay ingredients with a client.

and rejuvenation of mind, body and soul; on the other, it has roots in the country's rich source of indigenous, Malay, Indian and Chinese therapies. Sometimes, it offers a combination of modern technology with traditional ritual, thereby reflecting the diverse traditions of Malaysia's cultures.

Malaysia has a wide selection of spa options including destination spas, resort spas, hotel spas, cruise ship spas, day spas and medical spas. The settings for these run the gamut from luxury destinations and select hideaways to small establishments and individual practitioners' businesses. Some offer other Asian therapies, such as Thai and Balinese, as well.

Within the varying Asian traditions, some wellness customs (especially those of Chinese origin) are documented in ancient manuscripts, although there are countless medicinal formulations and recipes using herbs, spices, fruits and flowers that have been handed down orally from generation to generation. Developed in temples, palaces, monasteries or humble homes, they all encompass the knowledge that outer beauty comes from inner health. Their central tenet is balance.

The Malay Spa Today

A spa culture can be seen in ancient Malay healing practices, many of which incorporate the rejuvenating properties of water. Encompassing both beauty and medicine, these treatments were experienced in the rarefied environments of royal palaces as well as the courtyards of rural village homes. Beauty therapies included massage, body scrubs, scented body steaming, facial and hair treatments and baths, while medicinal therapies concentrated on feminine health, post-natal care and other gynecological and medical conditions. These drew on practices

Within the varying Asian traditions, some wellness customs are documented in ancient manuscripts.

Opposite Malay healing practices incorporate the rejuvenating properties of water.

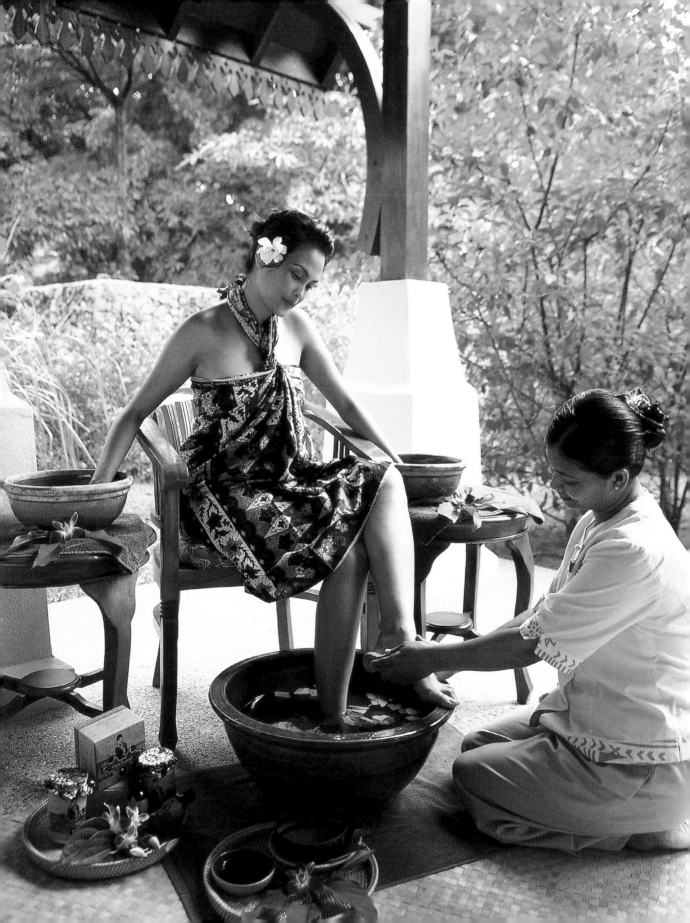

such as sitz baths, hot compresses, body wraps, herbal steaming and herbal baths.

A unique factor in Malay healing is that it places great emphasis on the wellness of the soul. Represented by the human reproductive system or *ujud anggota*, the soul is considered the life force of the human body. The ujud anggota is what differentiates a man from a woman and is seen as an indicator of the total wellbeing of the entire body. As such, it is integral in the drive to reduce the effects of aging.

Some Malay spas, mainly smaller concerns, incorporate completely genuine Malay treatments in their menus, but, more often than not, they absorb Western and other Asian traditions too. In certain instances, a few cutting-edge spas employ traditional healers to provide a highly authentic experience. Such cases involve the employment of *bidan* (midwives) or therapeutic masseurs who have received their skills from within the family. It's unusual to find such healers in world-class facilities, but it's believed that more are likely to make the transition from home to hotel, or private practice to international spa, in the future.

> A unique factor in Malay healing is that it places great emphasis on the wellness of the soul.

Malay Treatments: From the Forest to the Spa

So, what treatments is the guest likely to see on the Malay spa menu today? Drawing inspiration and ingredients from one of the oldest rainforests in the world and combining them with a legacy of multicultural healing, these therapies are a potent mix. Some remain resolutely authentic, while others incorporate elements from traditional Chinese medicine (TCM), Ayurveda and international sources.

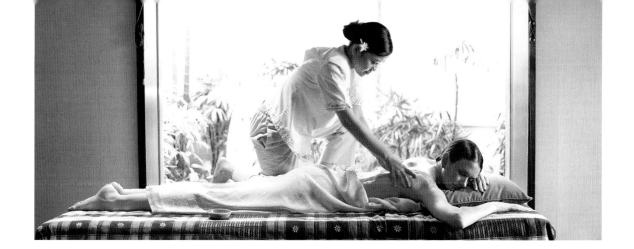

Malay Massage

Traditional Malay massage or *urut Melayu* varies from state to state and from one family to another. An oil massage, it mainly consists of long kneading strokes using thumb and palm pressure, although the use of elbows, edge of palm, arms and feet is also not uncommon. Urut Melayu is a deep tissue massage that focuses on the importance of the flow of blood in the *urat* or veins and arteries and normally starts from the feet and ends with a head and scalp massage. Strokes directed towards the heart (*buka urat*) invigorate, while strokes going away from the heart (*tutup urat*) are aimed at calming. Stretching exercises—for rejuvenation and anti-aging—are often the closing ritual.

Before the massage commences, the masseur or healer says a special *doa* or prayer for blessings on the therapy. He then acknowledges the four core elements of a human being, thus coaxing the body and its arteries, veins and nerves to settle into their original and perfect places before the massage commences.

Mainly aimed at stimulating energy points, loosening and warming up muscles and reducing aches, pains and flatulence, practitioners vary from midwives to *bomoh patah* (healers specializing in bone setting) to *tok guru silat* (silat masters). The bidan focuses on rejuvenation for the new mother, the bomoh patah specializes on the mending of bones and the tok guru silat works on increasing stamina and male virility.

Above An *urut Melayu* massage being performed.

Following pages Different techniques of *urut Melayu*, involving the use of elbows, palms, arms and feet.

Urut Melayu is a deep tissue massage that focuses on the importance of the flow of blood in the *urat* or veins and arteries and normally starts from the feet.

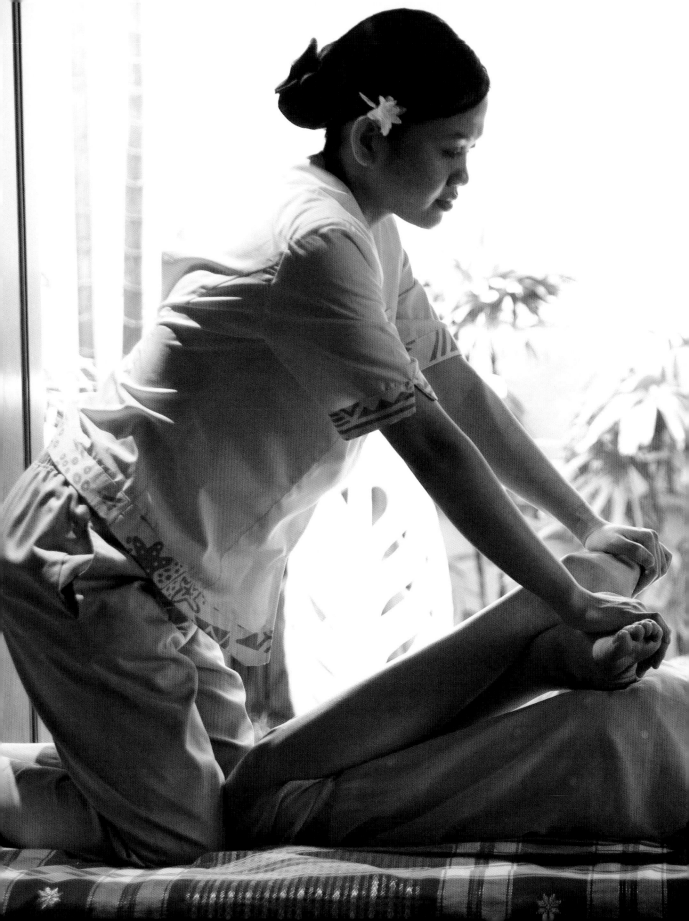

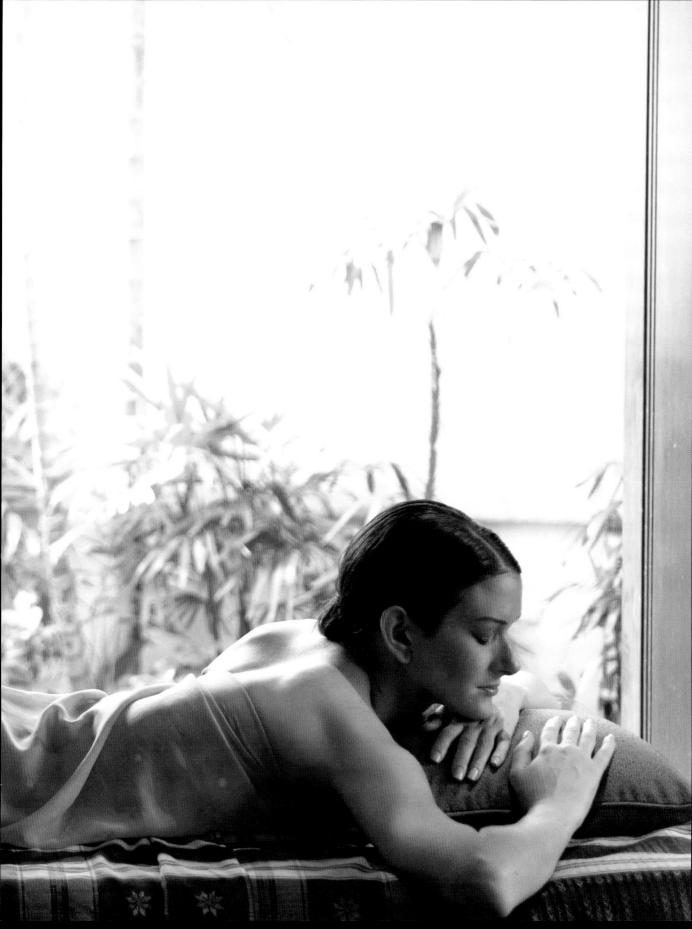

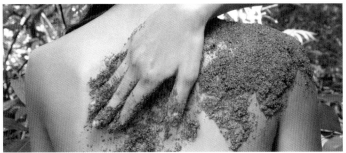

Herbal Body Scrubs

A scrub is an exfoliation that removes dead skin, dirt and debris from the skin's surface, all the while preparing it for better nutrient absorption. It also stimulates circulation and metabolism, helps eliminate waste and toxins from the lymphatic system, eases fluid retention and improves both skin texture and inner skin function. Often given prior to a wrap or steam bath, or as an essential pre-bathing cleansing ritual, its effectiveness lies in the skill of the therapist and the numerous components of the ingredients.

While the basic Malay recipe of ground rice, turmeric, nutmeg and galangal has become an industry standard, various other recipes have evolved. Warming scrubs include spices such as black pepper: these heat up the body, thereby reducing muscle and joint pains. There's something wonderfully nurturing about such a scrub, when the spicy scent of pepper mingles with the tingling of muscles. Another unique experience is the *gamat* or sea cucumber scrub. Recent research has revealed that sea cucumber accelerates the regeneration of cells, bone, collagen and skin, so this is an effective anti-aging scrub. And a scrub with the famed jungle tree *tongkat ali* is de rigeur: believed to relieve pain and itches, treat disease and enhance overall health, it is highly popular.

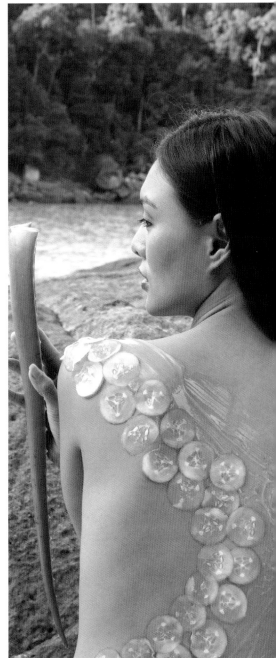

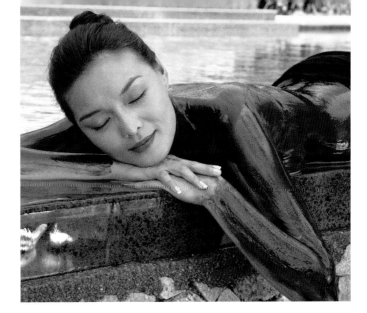

Body Masks

The Malay body mask or wrap has its origins in post-natal care. Warming herbs (such as betel, ginger, lemongrass and galangal) were favored as they induced sweating, thereby enhancing lymphatic drainage, detoxification and absorption of ingredients.

Many Malay spas offer traditional post-natal masks, but there has been much inventive adaptation. Banana leaves, plastic covers and thermal blankets have replaced cloth binders, and a multitude of different herbs, spices and plants are mixed for different results. Aloe vera, turnip and cucumber are used for cooling and nurturing, sea cucumber is a great healer and papaya is often applied for its enriching enzymes. Yoghurt, a skin soother and refresher, is also sometimes added to give extra nourishment.

Humble muds and marine compounds are increasingly making a name for themselves in the spa world too. Spas on the island of Borneo are known for their use of volcanic mud, therapeutic white clay, active marine ingredients and algae—all readily available locally. Known to draw out impurities, re-mineralize tissues, enrich blood, stimulate circulation and accelerate the elimination of toxins, they've been elevated to star status in spa circles in recent years.

Facial Therapies

Before the advent of pre-packaged lotions, potions and creams, most Malay facial products came from either the kitchen or the garden. Soaked rice water was used as a cleanser; turnip, lime or cucumber juices were toners; scrubs consisted of soaked rice pounded with turmeric; and masks were composed of rice pearls, clay, honey or egg.

Most spas are still using these natural ingredients today, a testament to the power of these homegrown treatments. Proving that the kitchen cosmetic never goes out of fashion, these basics are augmented with a variety of herbs or tropical fruits to further enhance skin regeneration, hydration and healing.

There's something wonderfully transporting about lying in splendid isolation in an ocean-side cabana or nurturing massage bed with the scents of freshly-mashed ingredients perfuming face and air. Knowing that the ingredients come straight from the market only heightens the experience.

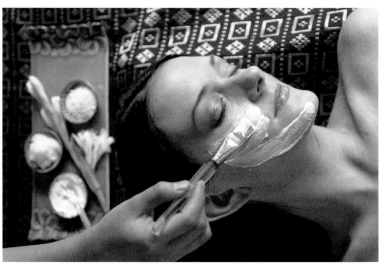

Above Traditional Malay facial products share many of the same ingredients as those used in the kitchen, such as turmeric, turnip and lime.

Right Masks are often applied with a brush, then left for 15 minutes to allow the ingredients to permeate the skin.

Opposite Facial products consist of scrubs, masks, toners, cleansers and more.

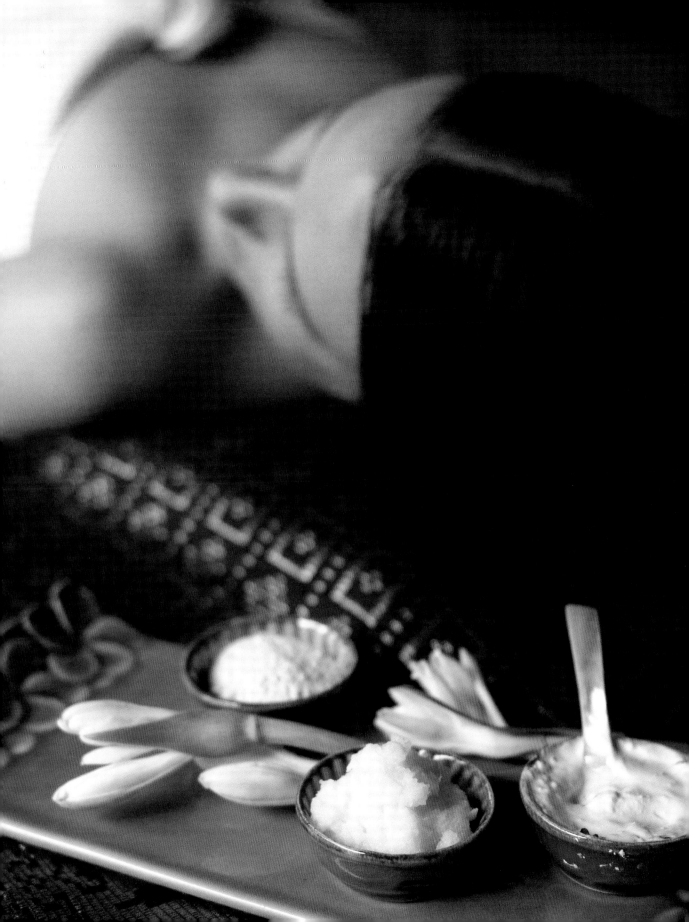

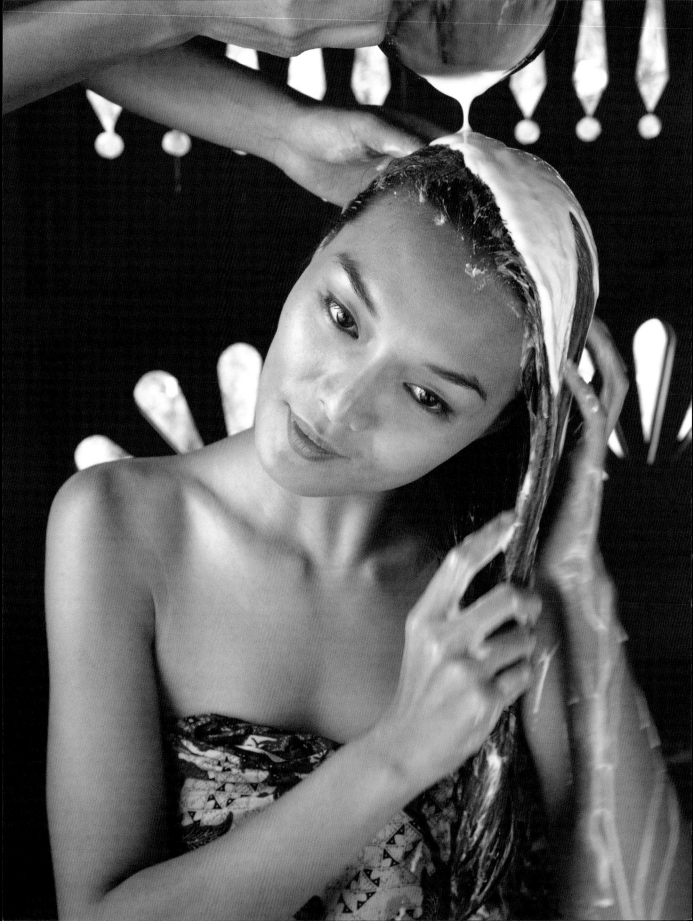

Hair Remedies

In Malaysia, as in other Asian countries, the coconut is the king of hair products. Traditionally, the oil was used to massage the scalp, stimulate circulation and strengthen hair roots, while the milk was reserved for conditioning.

Today, coconut milk is often used for hair conditioning rituals either alone or infused with essential oils or flowers. Hibiscus leaves and aloe vera are also popular conditioners, while sesame oil and candlenut (*Aleurites moluccana*) are alternatives for scalp massages. Some spas may offer a medicated recipe for relieving heat, migraines and dandruff: a powerful mix of betel and henna leaves, you can actually feel the heat being drawn out from the scalp!

Steam Baths

Sweat therapies form an integral part of Malay healing culture. Scented, beautifying steam therapies were part of bridal preparation rituals, while medicated steams were popular for post-natal and pre-natal health, as well as the enhancement of male virility and physique.

Body steaming or *ukup* was traditionally performed sitting on a special wooden stool with a small opening at its center; the treatment was believed to open up pores, release toxins, tone muscles and firm and smooth skin texture. Malays believe that ukup helps stabilize body temperature by balancing the four universal elements (earth, water, fire and wind). Whether this is true or not, a steam certainly eliminates body impurities through profuse sweating, breaks up stubborn fats and cellulite, alleviates sluggishness and clears the mind.

In Asia, coconut is the king of hair products. Coconut milk and oil are used to stimulate and strengthen the hair follicles in the scalp.

Opposite Coconut milk can be used either alone or infused with essential oils or flowers.

Below *Ukup wangi*, or fragrant sauna, ingredients.

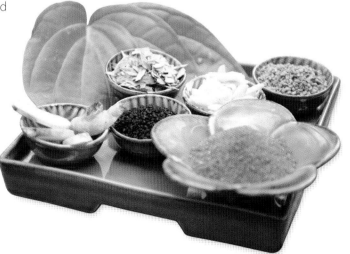

In modern spas, the traditional steaming method has largely been replaced by the use of sauna bags, sauna rooms and steam rooms. Clients can choose from a variety of options: *ukup wangi* or scented body steaming with infusions of pandan leaves, tropical blooms and splashes of fresh Kaffir lime is an uplifting cleansing experience. The spicy *ukup rempah*, used as a weekly therapy for Malay men or as a post-natal practice for women, is powerfully detoxifying, while many opt for the *ukup kering*, or dry herbal steam.

Hot Compresses

Often called *bertungku* and *bertuam* as *tungku* means 'the stone in a hearth' and *tuam* translates as a 'pain-reducing heated object wrapped with cloth and compressed on parts of the body', hot compresses are widely practiced in the Malay spa. Although originally enjoyed mainly by women in confinement after birth, nowadays men are increasingly becoming fans of these profoundly restorative experiences.

The *tungku batu*, an ancient but effective formulation from the Malay heritage, is a case in point. Typically, the body is vigorously rubbed with a medicated ointment of coconut oil, clove, nutmeg, galangal and lemongrass. Heated river or clay stones, wrapped with selected spices and herbs and tied in a cotton cloth, are then applied onto the body. The spices in the pouches often include fenugreek and black seed, and leaves such as betel and morinda (Indian mulberry). Renowned for its ability to relieve aches and pains, improve blood circulation and the functioning of the uterus, tungku batu also helps reduce cellulite and varicose veins. Spa guests have the added benefit of soothing, warming heat and the aroma of herbs and spices.

Below Hot compress, or *tungku batu*.

Opposite Hot compresses are popular with men as well as women.

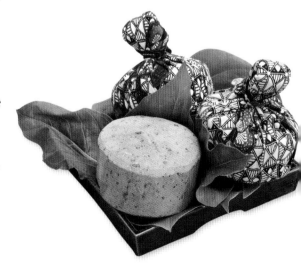

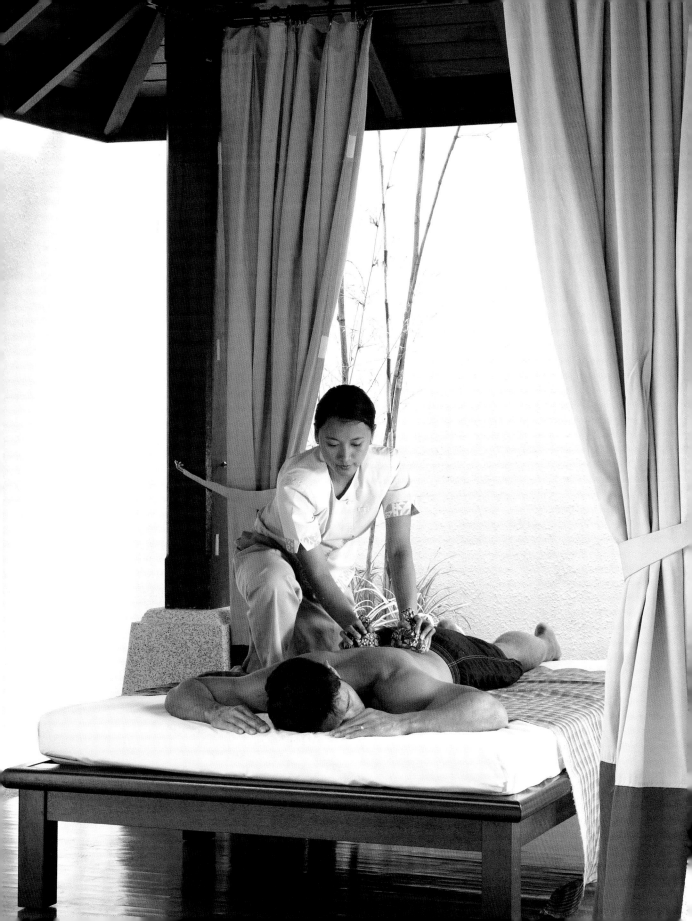

Herbal Teas

Long before the West brought the word 'detox' into the general lexicon, the Malays have been detoxing themselves every day with herbal drinks or *air akar kayu* and herbal concoctions such as *majun* and *julap*. Their uses are many: some are taken for specific reasons, such as weight loss or skin health, while others may be geared towards more general health benefits. Nonetheless, they all help to digest and absorb food efficiently, flush out waste products, aid liver function, eliminate toxins, reduce fat, blood sugar and cholesterol, and give the immune system a boost.

In line with the general spa trend of offering guests herbal beverages, most Malay spas offer pre- or post-treatment teas for a distinctively Malay experience.

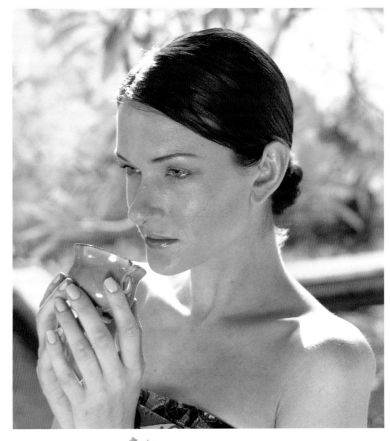

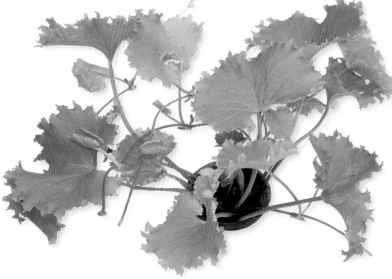

Infusions of *tongkat ali* or *kacip fatimah*, *pegaga* (*Centella asiatica*) or pandan, sweetened with honey, are fast gaining a loyal following. Pegaga tea (or *gotu kola* as it is known in the West) is believed to cleanse the blood, cure indigestion, nervousness and dysentery, and is a youth preservative. Its chemical constituents are reported to contain asiatic acid, asiaticoside, madecassic acid and madecassoside—certainly good for you and your skin (even if you aren't sure what they are!).

Opposite, above Herbal teas
have long been a tradition
and a way of life in Asia.

Opposite, below *Pegaga*,
a key ingredient in a Malay
herbal tea aimed at
enhancing youthfulness.

Below *Tuam pasir* is used on
joint pains and inflammations.

Another healing hot compress is the *tuam pasir*, traditionally used on joint pains, growths, severe inflammations and post-natal abdomens especially after a Caesarian section. Salt or sand is placed in a frying pan with fenugreek and black seed and cooked until hot. This concoction is then placed on a cotton cloth which is made into a pouch and used as a pressure massage. As with the tungku batu, a medicated ointment is applied first.

Malay Baths

Baths are an important aspect of spiritual and physical cleansing, and, as such, are an integral part of healing in the Malay tradition. In spas, such healing baths are often offered as a prelude or finale to another treatment.

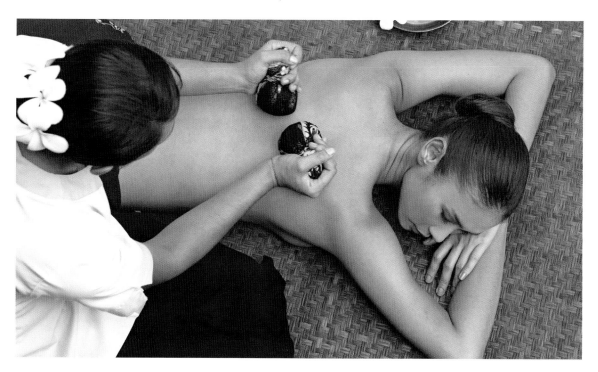

The variety is quite extraordinary with dozens of fruits, roots, leaves and flowers finding their way into enlivening, relaxing and healing waters. The uplifting floral bath, also widely found elsewhere in Asia, was a very popular practice in the courts of the Malay royal houses and is still practiced as a pre-wedding ritual (see page 54). Historically, one of the most important was the Malay lime bath. In ancient times only Kaffir lime and lime were used, but modern-day spas also add lemon and kalamansi as well as infusions of pandanus to enhance the aromatherapy effect. As lime is an astringent and an effective blood purifier, not to mention an all round detoxifier, the bath is believed to purge out illness, impurities and unwanted negative elements.

Jumping on to the thalassotherapy bandwagon, many spas—especially those in coastal areas—are now offering marine baths. Seawater is an age-old remedy for sore throats, arthritis, joint ailments, digestive problems and skin diseases. As it has the same chemical make-up as human plasma, seawater allows the body to absorb its mineral properties easily. Borneo sea salt and seaweed baths are often mixed with essential oils for a truly exotic, sensual experience.

Another powerful bath concoction—typically used for mothers in confinement and for conditions like arthritis, muscle aches and chills—consists of henna, betel leaves, black seed, sea salt, camphor, fenugreek and citronella tied together in a muslin cloth and boiled in a pot of water. Whether the concoction is added to the bath, placed on key parts of the body or used in a foot or sitz bath is at the discretion of the individual spa. When you inhale the strong herbal aroma, it awakens tired organs and boosts the body's lymphatic system. And when the properties from the herbs are absorbed into the system, muscles are conditioned and blood circulation improves.

Below Ingredients that make up the *sintok* bath.

Opposite This Malay floral bath uses Kaffir limes and flowers such as rose, jasmine and tuberose, creating a fragrant and refreshing infusion.

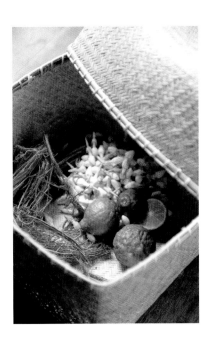

Fragrant Floral Bathing: A Rich Malay Tradition

The practice of bathing in waters suffused with the scents and healing properties of forest plants has been part of Malay tradition for hundreds of years. Formulated to calm and renew, impart energy, beautify or simply relax, such baths provide more than a physical cleansing experience. They're tied in with ideas of ritual purification of spirit and mind too.

The *mandi bunga puteri* or princess's floral bath has been practiced by girls in both the Malay royal courts and ordinary households for centuries. It was formulated as a ritual for girls reaching puberty or young women trying to attract desirable husbands. Using a number of fragrant and colorful blooms, the bath is believed to enhance facial glow and leave an enticing scent on the body. It is also thought to ward off negative elements both from within and without, imbuing the practitioner with a positive energy. It is now offered in beauty salons or may be self-administered.

The flowers are included in this princess's floral bath in odd-numbered quantities—such as five, seven or nine—and are combined with *akar sintok* (*Cinnamomum sintoc*) and Kaffir lime. In Malay tradition, lime is the tangible link to the forces of the spiritual world, so bathing in lime represents a symbolic relief of

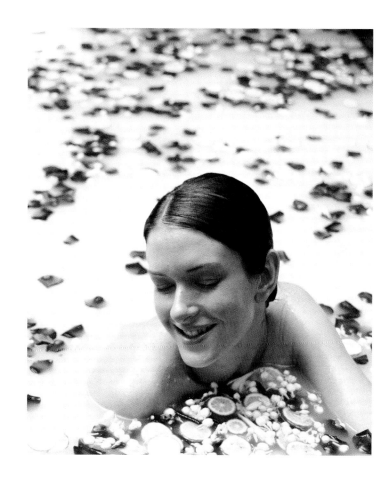

unwanted negative energies. Its zesty aroma and astringent properties combine with a high vitamin C content to cool the body and uplift the soul. Sintoc roots are cleansing and anti-bacterial as well as cooling on the body. The flowers may include: Jasmine (*Jasminum sambac*), rose (*Rosa* sp.), *kenanga* (*Cananga odorata*), *kesidang* (*Vallaris pergulana* Burm.*)*, *cempaka* (*Michelia champaca*) and *sundal malam* (*Polianthes tuberosa*).

After the petals have been separated and strewn in the bath, the lime and akar sintok are added for a long and soothing soak. The akar sintok may be rubbed onto the scalp to strengthen hair roots and prevent dandruff and excess heat, while the Kaffir lime can be mashed onto the scalp to promote glossy hair. The overall effect should be hydrating, aroma-therapeutic, refreshing and purifying—and when a handsome prince then walks through the door, so much the better!

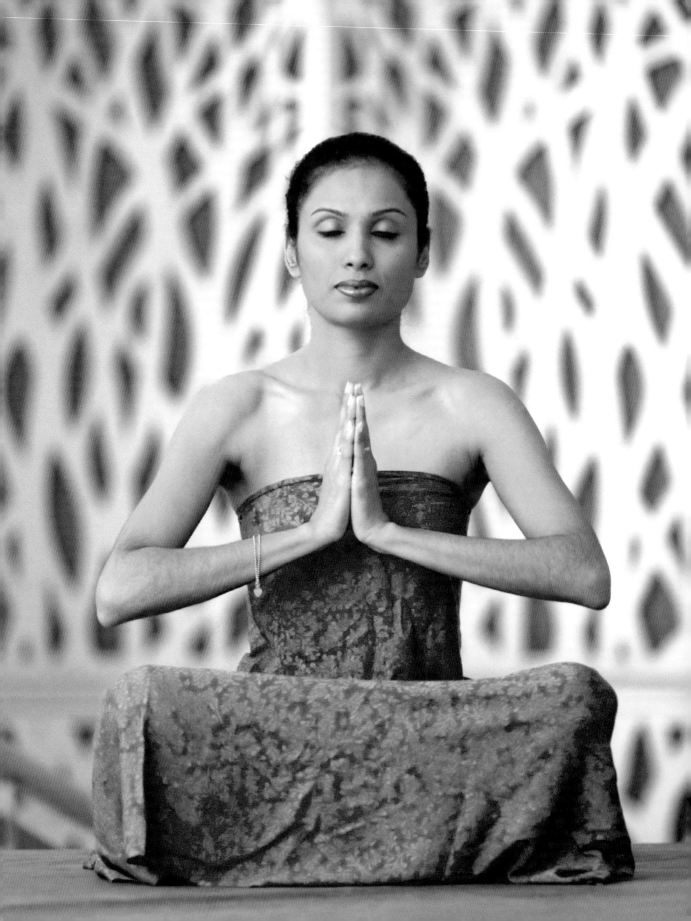

The Ayurvedic Spa

Malaysia's long history of Ayurveda has been one of local and family use, with Ayurvedic methods for promoting health and managing common ailments part of the daily routines of Indian families in Malaysia (see pages 130–149). Ayurvedic treatments also appear to have had an early influence on the home-care routines of Malays.

While water has been the key element in Western spas since Roman times, it is oil that is the essential element in the Ayurvedic rejuvenating regime. Oleation, as it is termed by Ayurvedic doctors, was far more central in the historic antecedents of the Ayurvedic spa than was water, although steam has an important role in eliminating toxins through the skin.

In most parts of the world, what we now call the Ayurvedic spa has its roots in the Ayurvedic clinic. In India, these are run by *vaidyas* or Ayurvedic physicians and offer both outpatient and residential care. In the latter category, one of the best-known in-house programs is the *panchakarma* regimen. A detoxifying course that focuses on rejuvenation and revitalization, it has five (*panch*) main actions (*karma*); depending on the patient's body type, one, two, three, four or five of these may be administered over a two- to six-week period (see page 206).

This classical form of Ayurvedic rejuvenation is now making its way into spas throughout Asia, along with a few other Ayurvedic options. In recent years, a number of Ayurveda-themed spas have emerged in Kuala Lumpur, Langkawi and elsewhere in Malaysia, drawing in varying degrees on these classical and clinical origins. Some have resident Ayurvedic physicians, while others draw on Indian practices and combine them with other Asian disciplines.

Panchakarma, which means five (*panch*) main actions (*karma*), is a detoxifying course that focuses on rejuvenation and revitalization.

Opposite The Ayurvedic spa has its roots in the Ayurvedic clinic.

On the Menu

Ayurvedic spas in Malaysia tend to have short menus with a variety of oil massages, some steam therapies and *sirodhara*, a therapy that involves oiling the 'third eye' (see pages 205–206). The emphasis is on one-off relaxation and rejuvenation, rather than a program to restore deep balance at the level of tissues. In addition, some Ayurvedic centers (more clinics than spas) have emerged offering panchakarma.

Recently, there are fresh initiatives being undertaken by the local authorities to establish Ayurvedic departments in a few select hospitals and there are plans to license some full clinical programs in Ayurveda. Undoubtedly, there will be some trickle-down effect in the country's spas in the decades to come. In the meantime, expect to see some of the following on the menu.

Abhyanga Massage

Although the etymology of the word *abhyanga* is disputed, most Ayurvedic physicians hold that the word translates as 'massage against the direction of hairs'. It is a stimulating rather than soothing experience, and enhances the activity of the microcirculatory system in the skin. Abhyanga is traditionally performed with a medicated herbal oil chosen according to one's *dosha* (principles of physiology), and is performed by one, two, four, or more therapists simultaneously.

Long strokes, mainly with full palm involved, in the direction of blood circulation from the trunk to the extremities and up to down, are employed. Reverse hand movements are passive (without pressure). As the oil is massaged into the body, its healing, stimulating (or other) properties are absorbed into the system via the skin.

Opposite During the *abhyanga* massage, long strokes in the direction of blood circulation from the trunk to the extremities are employed.

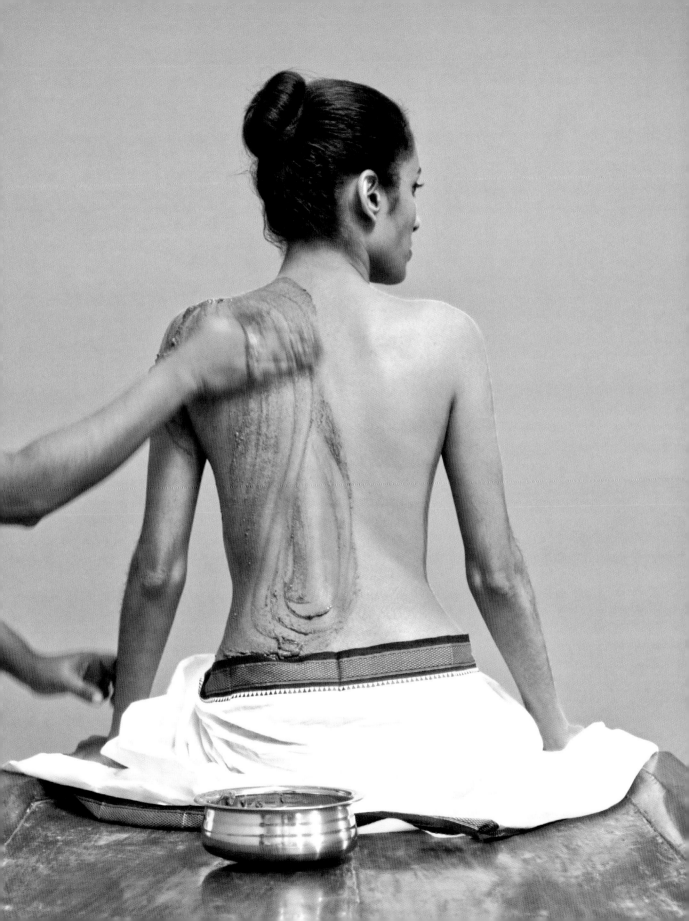

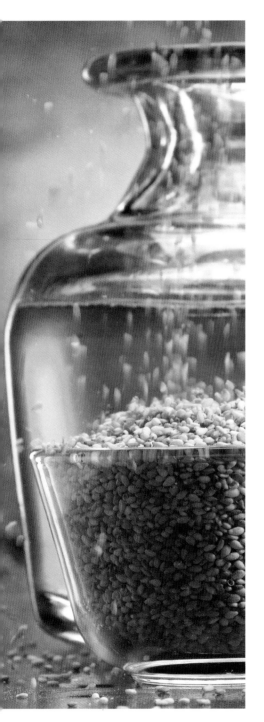

Ayu's Story: Ayurveda in the Home

While not clinical in origin, Ayurvedic spa rituals in Malaysia have deep cultural roots in the family, one of which is the practice of taking regular sesame oil baths. Ayu, a Malaysian from an Indian family, recalls his boyhood in the 1960s in the rural state of Pahang: 'Every few Saturdays, our parents would give us an oil bath. Whether we wanted it or not, it was

The 'home spa' oil bath is a typical component of the healthcare regimes practiced by many Indian families in Malaysia. Their daily (*dinacharya*) and seasonal (*ritucharya*) routines regularly included such practices.

a family tradition and we had to go along with it. We would sit outside, under a tree, while our mother or father would bathe and massage us with gingelly (sesame) oil. We'd let the oil soak in and, after a while, take an afternoon nap—the most restful sleep you can imagine! We'd feel so refreshed and clean when we woke up and our skin would be glowing.'

Illustrating the family commitment to this routine is an old Indian family saying: 'Instead of paying heavy fees to the doctor, pay a small sum regularly to the oil-seller and keep fit.' The massage oil used by Ayu's family was extracted locally using a wooden press or stone grinder. This yielded cold pressed oil that is a natural antioxidant, dense in nutrients and high in polyunsaturated fatty acids. The oil was stored in large clay pots and left exposed to direct sunlight in the open courtyard for a full day or two before being stored indoors.

Unknown to Ayu, sesame oil has anti-bacterial, anti-fungal, anti-viral and anti-inflammatory properties and was an effective treatment for the teenage acne that some of his friends were afflicted by. The exposure to sunlight after extraction allowed the oil to absorb vitamin D and hence convey it trans-dermally during the massage.

Ayu's 'home spa' oil bath is a typical component of the healthcare regimes practiced by many Indian families in Malaysia. Their daily (*dinacharya*) and seasonal (*ritucharya*) routines, inherited from their parents and grandparents, regularly included such practices. Today, because Ayurvedic clinics and hospitals are still relatively few, these time-honored family healthcare traditions form much of the inspiration for Ayurvedic spas in modern-day Malaysia.

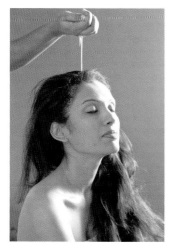
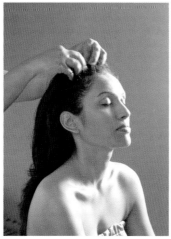

Indian Head Massage

This revitalizing massage involves work not only on the head but on the upper back, shoulders, neck, scalp and face too. In much the same way that TCM dictates that certain points on the feet are directly aligned to internal organs, Ayurveda holds that certain parts of the head are related to other body parts and symptoms or diseases. Therefore, a *champi* or head massage does not only affect the immediate areas massaged: it can be a healing, rejuvenating and thoroughly stimulating experience as well.

The massage is usually given seated in a chair and may be dry or with nourishing oils to condition hair and calm the nervous system. The therapist usually starts by gently kneading upper back, shoulder and neck muscles, then works up to the head. Here, the scalp is squeezed, rubbed and tapped and hair may be combed or pulled. Key pressure or *marma* points (similar to acu-points in TCM) are attended to, and the session ends with a facial massage that mixes acupressure and gentle manipulation with soft stroking.

Opposite Sesame oil has anti-bacterial, anti-fungal, anti-viral and anti-inflammatory properties.

Far left *Champi*, or head massage, may be given either dry or with nourishing oils.

Left The scalp is squeezed, rubbed and tapped during an Indian head massage.

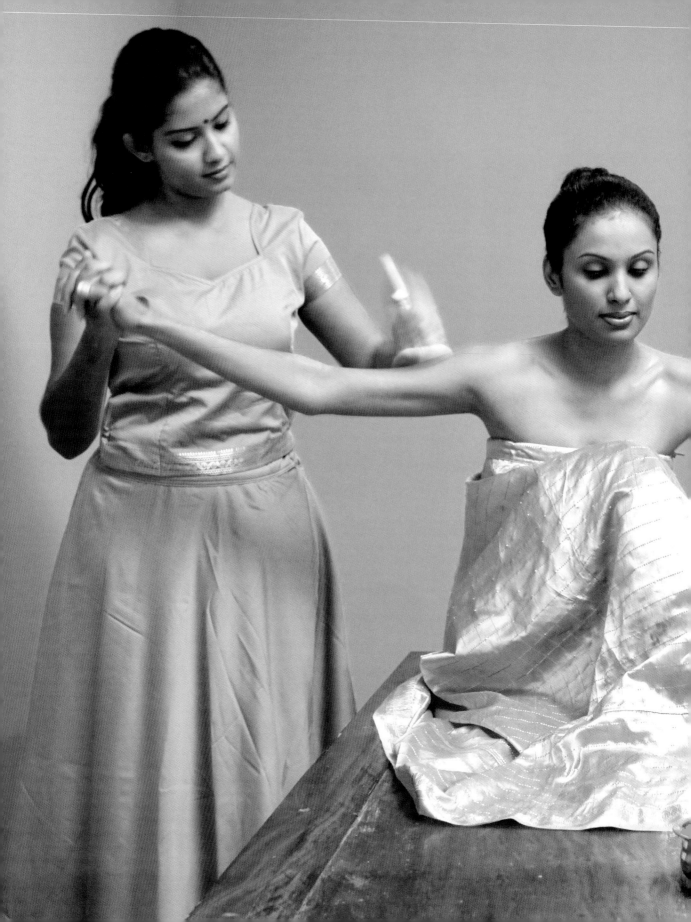

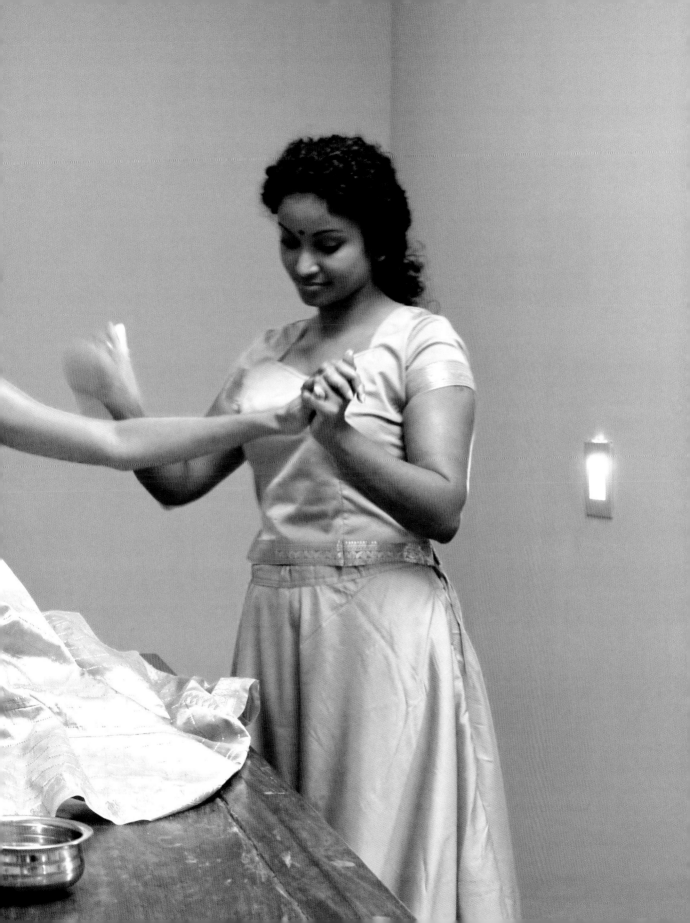

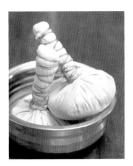

Previous pages Herbal pouches used in *swedanam* usually contain leaves from plants, such as the drumstick tree and castor oil plant.

Above right *Abhyanga* literally means 'against the direction of the hairs', making it a stimulating massage experience.

Above left Herbal pouches.

Below The fast movements of the herbal pouch massage are also smooth and warm, giving the experience of deep relaxation.

Opposite, above A Mughal painting of a *ghulam*, or bath attendant, attending to a customer in a traditional bath house.

Opposite, below Ayurvedic facials work on inner and outer levels of the skin.

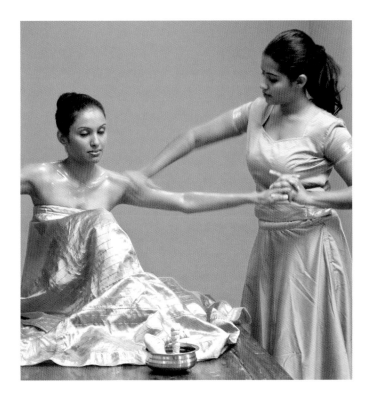

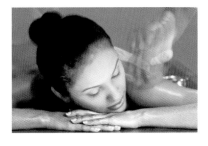

Herbal Pouches

Classified as a *swedanam* (sweat therapy) in the Vedic texts, the herbal poultice is a time-honored detoxifying and healing tradition. Not unlike the Malay practice of healing with heated compresses, specially selected ingredients are tied tightly in natural cloth, steamed for a few minutes, then dipped in medicated herbal oil and applied to the body. On application, the heat induces sweating, thereby helping to eliminate toxins via the skin's surface; then, once the pores are open, the skin absorbs the properties of the herbs for healing.

A variety of different plants are used in the pouches, but expect to see leaves from the castor oil plant (*Ricinus communis*), *Datura alba* leaves, skin tonifying *lemuni* (*Vitex*

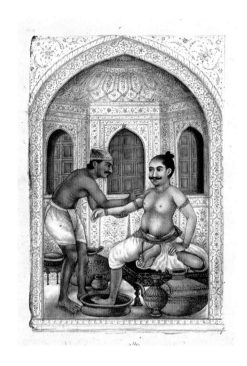

negundo) and leaves from the drumstick tree (*Moringa oleifera*). The latter are a well-known natural antibiotic, but all these leaves contain anti-inflammatory and pain-reducing properties, so are useful for arthritic conditions. Mixed with crushed garlic, lime and shredded coconut flesh and fried with medicated oil in an earthen or clay pan, they penetrate deeply into the subcutaneous layers of the skin.

Facial and Hair Treatments

A number of Ayurvedic beauty treatments utilizing herbal facial and hair care products are offered in Malaysian Indian-themed spas. Hair washes use such plants as vetiver, *tulsi* (holy basil) and acacia, or neem and *gotu kola* (*Centella asiatica*). Traditionally, Indians washed their hair with powder, not shampoo, as powder doesn't strip the hair of its natural oils. Coconut milk is often used for conditioning afterwards.

A variety of facials to condition and nourish skin, open blocked pores, eliminate toxins and cleanse the face are also offered. Therapeutic neem or 'the pharmacy tree' features prominently in such offerings, as do a variety of tropical fruits and vegetables, such as cooling cucumber and carrot. The underlying principle of all Ayurvedic facials is to work on both the inner and outer levels of the skin in order to develop *ojas* (see page 138). If ojas is strong and healthy, one has a radiant inner self; this, in turn, manifests itself in one's outer physical appearance.

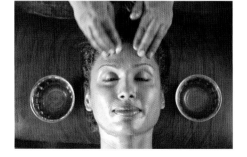

Sirodhara

Coming from *siro* ('head') and *dhara* ('pouring of herbal liquids on specific body parts'), sirodhara comprises the continuous

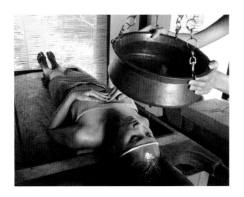

pouring of herbal oils, milk, buttermilk or ghee over the head and scalp. The client lies on his or her back on a wooden treatment table, cocooned in warm towels, while a therapist trains a steady rhythmic stream of warm liquid from a perforated vessel made of clay, wood or metal on to the forehead.

Oil stroking the forehead and the underlying frontalis muscle has a balancing effect on the deepest recesses of the brain and is profoundly relaxing. In Ayurveda, it is seen as a stimulating procedure and is used in conjunction with other therapies for specific medicinal conditions. Its recent inclusion in spas is less therapeutic in nature and more relaxing. During a session, the nervous system unwinds, the busy brain becomes clear, and the tired body is refreshed.

Above Herbal oils, milk, buttermilk or ghee can be used in *sirodhara*.

Below Ayurvedic herbalized steam baths open the pores and allow toxins to be eliminated through the skin.

Opposite In clinics, *sirodhara* is used in conjunction with other therapies for specific medicinal conditions.

Panchakarma

While Ayurveda is known to have existed in India and neighboring countries for some thousands of years, the concept of 'spa' has only recently been applied to the age-old Ayurvedic rejuvenation system known as *panchakarma*. *Panch* means 'five' in Sanskrit and *karma* means 'action'. Panchakarma, therefore, refers to the five principle therapeutic strategies or actions employed in Ayurvedic rejuvenation.

Offered at a few forward-thinking spas in Malaysia, the process is deeply detoxifying and restores balance to the physiology, comprising an individual program of medication, diet, treatments

and more. After intensive consultation with an Ayurvedic physician, the five-pronged treatment usually follows three stages: *purvakarma* or preparation, *pradhanakarma* or treatments, and *paschatkarma* or post-treatment care.

Preparatory procedures are designed to help the body discard toxins present in the stomach and tissues and help facilitate their movement to the alimentary canal, then, when the body and mind are deemed ready, pradhanakarma or the main treatment designed to each individual's needs, begins.

Panchakarma is a profound procedure, so it is usually followed by post-treatment care as well. Levels of

doctor/patient trust need to be strong, the client needs to stay focused, and enough time must be set aside for what can be a deep inner journey. Many people report that it is a life-changing experience. It should be noted, also, that some spas offer differing forms of panchakarma programs. It is worth doing some research before embarking on the journey.

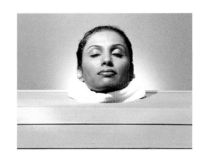

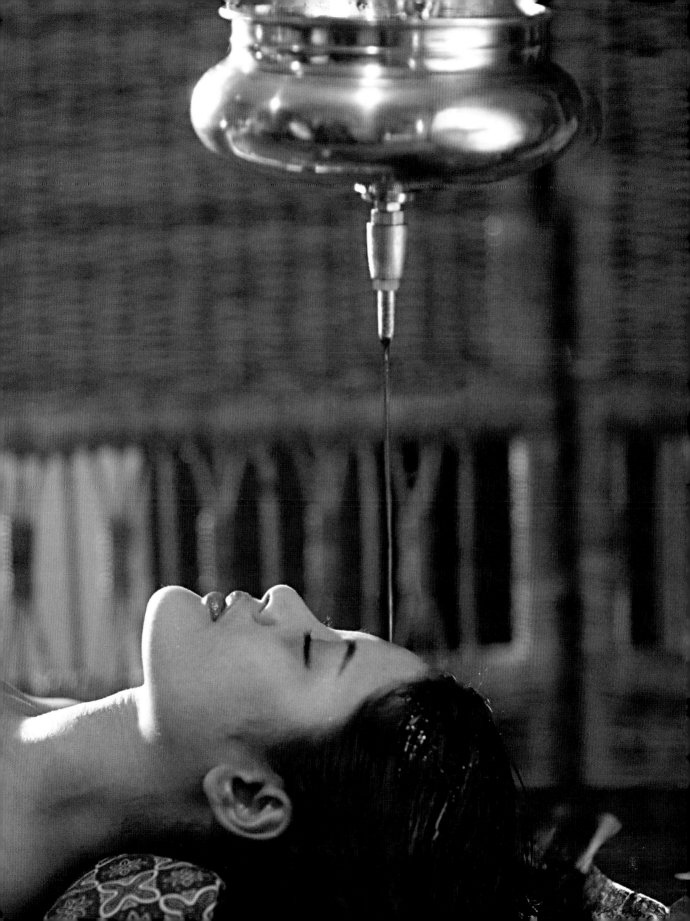

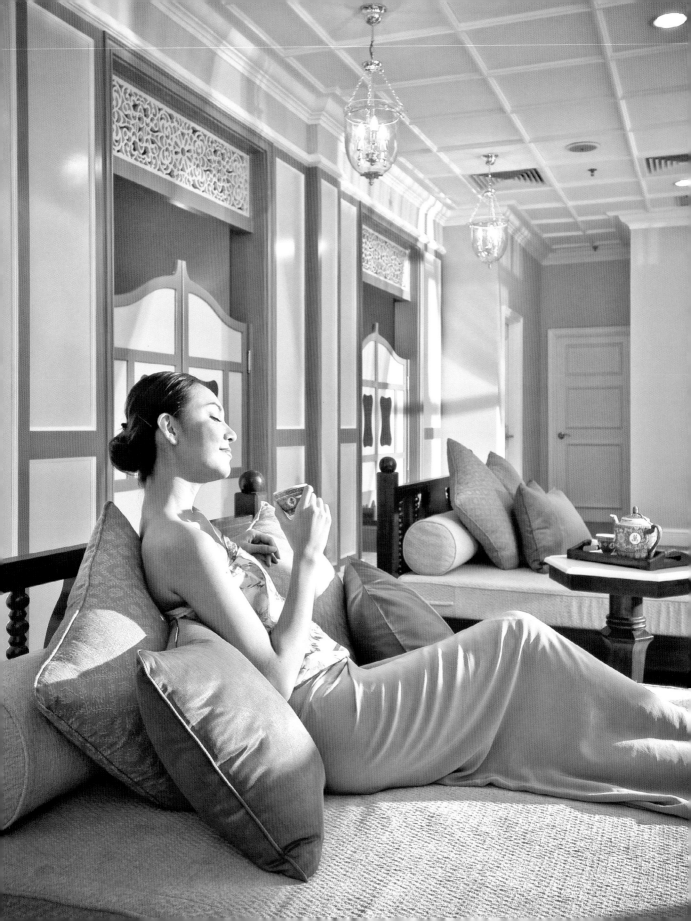

We now see a smattering of herbal wellness rituals taken from the Peranakan culture as well as a resurgence in popularity of cooling teas, nourishing soups and herbal cuisine regularly consumed by Malaysian Chinese households.

Opposite Peranakan Chinese-themed spas are a perfect example of traditional wisdom adapted to suit modern society.

Traditional Chinese Medicine (TCM) and Spa Culture

In modern Malaysian spa settings, you'll often find some Chinese or TCM-based wellness therapies on the menu. Unlike other spa cultures, these treatments are rarely water-based, as TCM did not favor specific therapies that utilized the healing properties of water. Certainly there was hot-spring bathing in China, with physicians acknowledging its therapeutic value particularly in the treatment of skin problems and joint pain, but for the most part such bathing was reserved for royalty.

Hands-on therapies—massage, reflexology, acupuncture, moxabustion and cupping—all derived from standard TCM are fairly common. The inclusion of a number of beauty treatments that take their inspiration from the archives of China's Imperial court physicians is perhaps more surprising, but then again, beauty products made from pearl powder, green tea and ginseng have been used by Malaysian Chinese for centuries.

In addition, taking the step from home to spa, we now see a smattering of herbal wellness rituals taken from the Peranakan culture as well as a resurgence in popularity of cooling teas, nourishing soups and herbal cuisine regularly consumed by Malaysian Chinese households.

It's encouraging to see this traditional wisdom gaining credence and popularity in Malaysia's spa world. An afternoon's session involving a facial derived from the Imperial court followed by a healing TCM reflexology session and foot bath, with perhaps a Peranakan hair treatment thrown in for good measure, is now a genuine option. Premium resort operators have tapped into TCM and Malaysia's rich cultural heritage to create Chinese-themed award-winning spas.

On the Menu

Such forward-thinking spas are increasingly trying to widen their appeal by integrating genuine TCM and Chinese-inspired therapies into their menus. So what are these therapies? One of the most important features of TCM is the regular flow of *qi* or life force, so a number of manual therapies that encourage this are found in TCM spas. According to TCM theory, while qi gives direction and support to blood flow, it is blood that generates qi. The art of massage, acupuncture, moxabustion and cupping manipulates the flow of qi and blood by using external aids—hands, needles, lit moxa sticks and suction cups respectively.

Massage

TCM massage is the most prevalent hands-on therapy found in spas. Called *an-mo* ('press and rub') or *tui-na* ('push and hold'), it has evolved throughout the centuries into many different styles with numerous variations of hand techniques. In principle, TCM massage seeks to achieve two important therapeutic outcomes—tonifying (strengthening) or sedating (relaxing) the body and mind. A light touch on specific acu-points for a short period of time generally produces a strengthening benefit, thereby increasing warmth and settling 'wind' in the body. A harder rub, again on specific acu-points but for a longer period of time, tends to give a relaxing benefit, with a general outcome of lightness (dampness removed) and cooling.

In the Malaysian spa, TCM massage is primarily offered as a means of relaxation and stress reduction, so techniques tend towards the harder, deeper rubs and kneads on specific areas of the body. For those who sit at the computer for long periods of time and have stiff shoulders and necks, a tui-na session for an hour or so can be a perfect way to ease away these tensions.

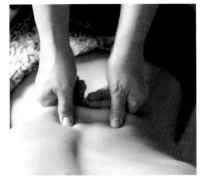

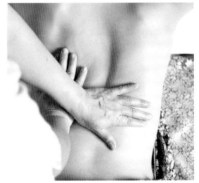

Top The *na* (grasping) technique.

Above The *an* (pressing) technique employed in *tui-na* massage.

Opposite *Tui-na* may be applied on face and neck, using one or two hands.

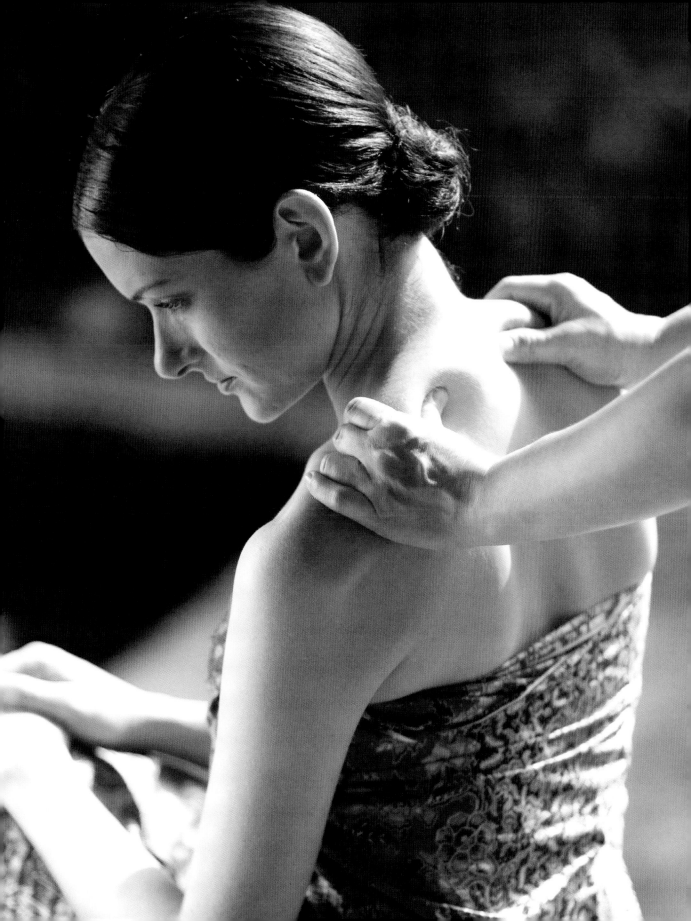

Cooling Teas, Nourishing Soups and Herbal Cuisine

One of the long-standing lifestyle health practices of the Chinese is the regular consumption of cooling teas, nourishing soups and herbal dishes. Finding themselves in an extremely hot and humid country, the Chinese population in Malaysia has sought to counteract minor health imbalances from excessive heat and dampness (excessive sweating, dry throats, extreme thirst, headaches and loss of appetite) via herbal self-care.

Simple herbal brews such as infusions of honeysuckle blooms and licorice root help in alleviating sore and itchy throats, while green tea and peppermint relieve minor headaches after sun exposure. Herbs used in cooling teas perform the function of reducing heat and dampness and the majority of them tend to be bitter. In order to enhance palatability, rock sugar is often added to these concoctions.

The majority of savory soups, on the other hand, tend to be nourishing or strengthening. A handful of wolfberries and five cloves were brewed in a pot to nourish *qi* and blood. Mutton with astragalus root and red dates with pinches of spices like fenugreek, fennel, alpinia seeds, allium seeds and cinnamon made a potent soup to strengthen *yin* (fluids) and *yang* (hormones), enhancing virility and improving fertility and strength.

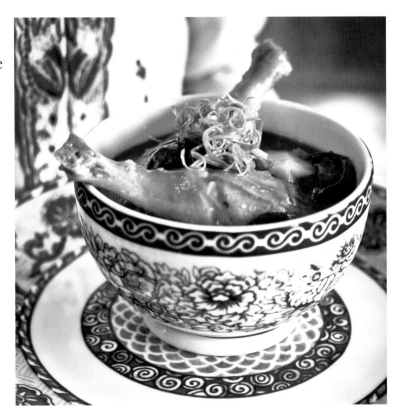

The creativity of Chinese cuisine comes into play when herbs are incorporated into delicious and healthy dishes going beyond teas and soups. From a TCM perspective, all foods are medicinal, so herbal desserts are often consumed both for taste and health benefit. They run the gamut from simple (steamed pears with apricot kernels and honey for a chronic dry cough) to time-consuming and luxurious. Double-boiled premium bird's nest with ginkgo nuts and rock sugar falls into the latter category.

The time-tested efficacy of Chinese teas, soups and cuisine has been capitalized on by a handful of Malaysian spas. With the right presentation, reasonable health claims and further fine-tuning, the potential for these drinks and dishes to globalize is unlimited. At present, they are offered as adjuncts to treatments in a small percentage of establishments—but they're sure to become more prevalent in the future.

Above Savory soups tend to be nourishing and strengthening.

Opposite Herbal teas have different functions, depending on the types of herbs used.

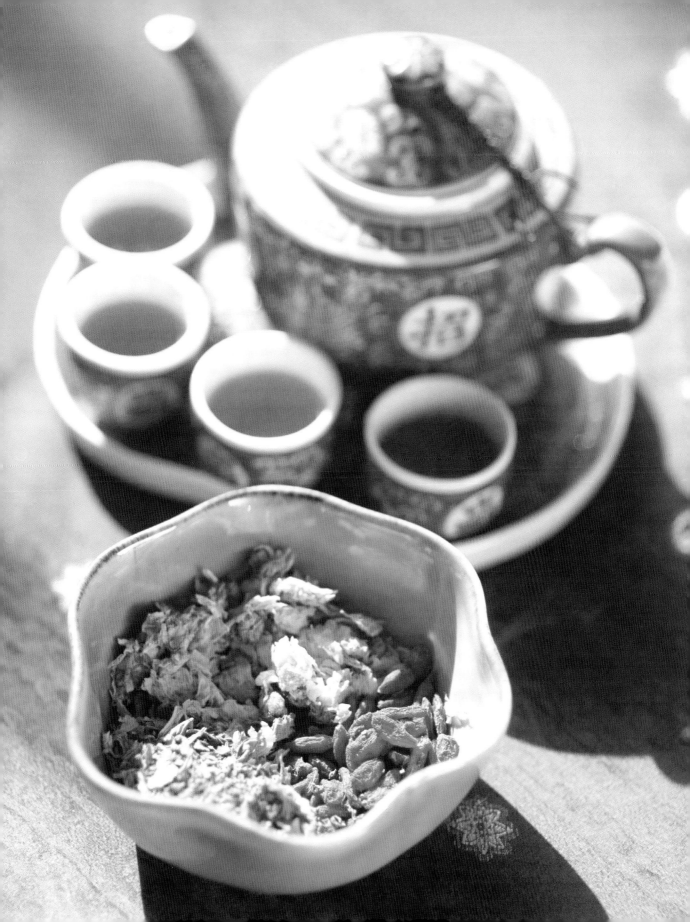

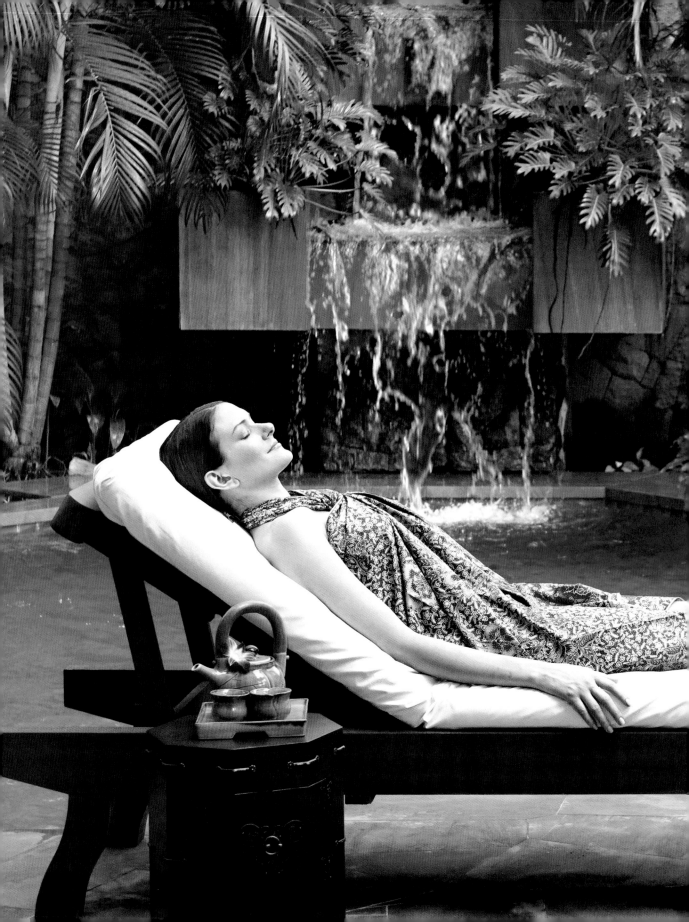

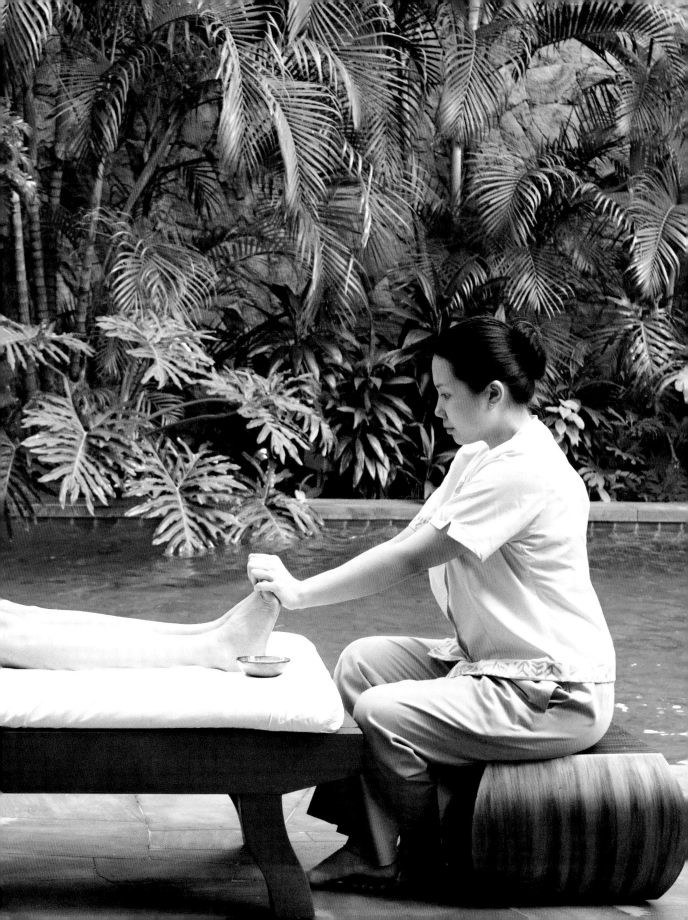

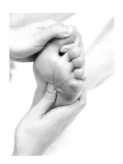

A foot reflexology session is as ubiquitous at a luxury spa (as here) as it is in shopping malls and smaller outlets all over Malaysia.

Above Foot reflexology works on specific areas. For example, the toes are believed to correspond to the head.

Below Moxa sticks, when rotated around areas of the body, encourage the flow of *qi*.

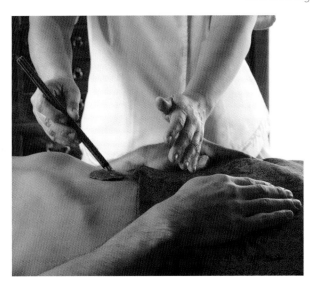

Reflexology

Hand and foot reflexology is another popular option. TCM advocates that specific areas of the hands and feet correspond to specific organs and functions of the body, so work on specific areas delivers therapeutic outcomes on specific organs. For example, the toes are believed to correspond to the head, so pressure-point massage on the toes may help relieve headache and neck tension. Many spa guests simply luxuriate in an invigorating foot massage for its own enjoyment, but if there are therapeutic internal benefits as well, so much the better!

Moxabustion

In essence, moxabustion advocates the placement of burning aromatic moxa leaves (*Artemesia vulgaris*) on acu-points to treat dampness and cold-induced complaints like chronic joint aches, asthma in the elderly and a variety of children's health complaints. There are two prevailing methods: non-scarring and scarring. Although most clients prefer the former for obvious cosmetic reasons, within the inner circle of moxa practitioners, almost everyone agrees that the scarring technique produces faster and more effective therapeutic outcomes.

Moxabustion is gaining popularity in resort spa settings where open-air space is easily available, but can be a challenge in spas with limited space as the aroma of the burning moxa plant can be overwhelming. On the other hand, it is important to note that moxabustion's efficacy does not only come from the heat, but also from the inhalation of the aroma of the burning plant.

An Empress's Regime: From Past to Present

In the late 19th century, the Empress Dowager Cixi's treatment program read like the menu of a particularly exotic spa ritual. Suffering from poor health since her youth, she frequently complained of poor vision, dryness and occasional itchiness of the eyes. Her physicians attributed this to excess heat and dampness in the liver, so came up with a number of remedies:

:: **Chrysanthemum Longevity Syrup:** Fresh chrysanthemum leaves were boiled then further reduced and mixed with honey. This syrup was taken daily with hot water.

:: **Eye-Brightening Remedy:** A powder—made by grinding 10 ingredients including mulberry leaves, chrysanthemum flowers, antelope horn shavings and oyster shell—was mixed with honey and turned into small pills. Several pills were taken daily.

:: **Brightening Vision Snuff:** Ten herbs including peppermint, rhubarb and camphor were all ground into fine powder and put in a snuff bottle. The empress was encouraged to inhale the powder especially on hot days or when she felt congestion in her eyes.

:: **Mulberry Leaf Eyewash:** Several mulberry leaves were boiled and the water was used to wash the eyes daily.

:: **Foot Bath to Eliminate Dampness:** Licorice, philodendron bark and chaenomeles fruit, along with five

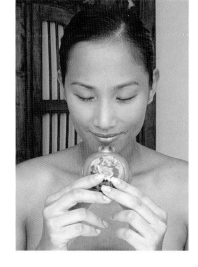

other herbs, were boiled in water and the decoction was used by the empress in a non-windy room as a foot soak.

Such remedies are now being analyzed and researched by TCM doctors and spa therapists, and some of the more adventurous Malaysian spas are beginning to offer similar treatments, but in a modern spa setting. After all, only a few minor modifications are needed to re-work the Empress Dowager Cixi's program into a fresh and inspiring spa ritual. Relief of stress, a general feeling of wellbeing and an alleviation of 'dampness' would leave clients refreshed and rejuvenated, for sure.

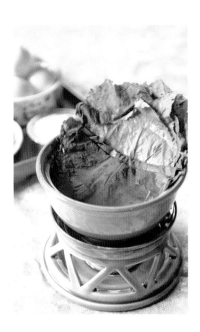

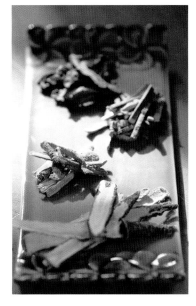

Above Brightening vision snuff.
Far left Mulberry leaf eyewash.
Left Herbs used in foot bath.

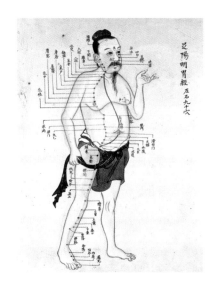

Acupuncture

Acupuncture is considered the most invasive but, at the same time, the most comprehensive therapy amongst TCM's basic hands-on treatments. A skilled acupuncturist can attend to acute and chronic problems, strengthen and sedate the system, as well as harmonize the body and mind by reducing excesses of cold, heat, dryness, dampness, 'wind' or 'scorching fire'. Thin, disposable needles are used to pierce specific acu-points in the body, and are generally retained for 20 to 30 minutes in most standard treatments. When pierced, a numbing, sore sensation on or around the point is considered a desirable therapeutic response.

In the hands of skillful acupuncturists, sharp pain is not experienced, but certain acu-points, especially those at the limbs' extremities are particularly sensitive and vulnerable to pain. Due to this and the invasive nature of the therapy, acupuncture is only offered in a very few specialist TCM spas in Malaysia.

Cupping

An unusual therapy, cupping is generally employed for heat-induced and 'wind' related problems such as chronic tension headache and hypertension. In its original form, the horns of animals were placed on specific acu-points of the body after they had been exposed to a flame source that created air pressure suction within. Today, special plastic or glass cups with an opening and hand-held pump are generally used by TCM doctors. The pump is operated manually to create the suction required.

The most common area where the cups are placed is on the lower abdomen and back along the sides of the spine.

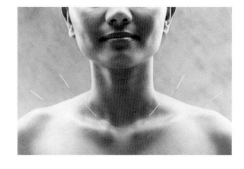

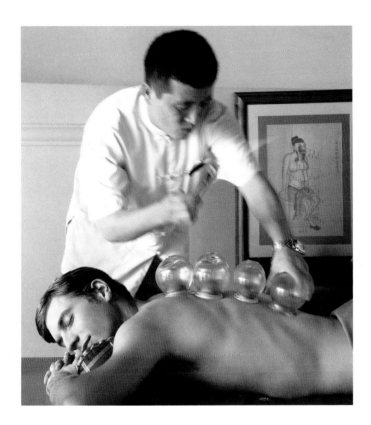

The suction formed in the cup pulls or sucks up the skin, forming a strong lump. Within a few seconds, with the ongoing suction, the surface of the lump starts to turn red, and in some cases, due to the bursting of minute capillaries on the skin's surface, purple. The cups are left in place for five to 15 minutes, but after removal leave red, circular patches that generally disappear after three days or so.

Areas of tightness, perceived as stagnation in TCM, are also deemed appropriate for cupping; the more serious the stagnation, the deeper the color of the marked patch. Because cupping is considered stress-relieving, the practice is gaining ground in Malaysian TCM-themed spas.

Opposite, above Painting of a male figure marked with acupuncture points.

Opposite, below Acupuncture is widely accepted as a form of pain relief.

Left Cupping is helpful in relieving joint stiffness and pain.

Below Red, circular patches appear after the removal of the cups.

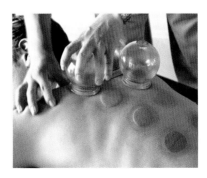

Peranakan Rituals

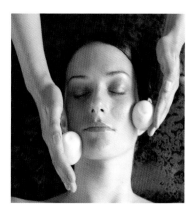

Based on the Chinese belief that true wellbeing is the product of a healthy balance of *yin* and *yang* (dark and light, cold and hot), Peranakan rituals made their global debut at a beautiful spa in Melaka in early 2008. Designed by a TCM doctor and taking their inspiration from home remedies used in Peranakan households, the signature rituals are intriguingly named *suam-suam panas* experience and *shiok-shiok sejuk* experience. Roughly translating as 'warming heat' experience and 'cool cold' experience respectively, they each involve a highly unusual sequence.

Upon arrival at the spa, guests are asked to fill in a questionnaire that determines whether they are predominantly a cool or warm person. This includes enquiries on health of skin, temperature, digestion and sleep patterns. The guests' answers allow the therapist to ascertain whether the client would benefit most from

a warming or cooling experience. After diagnosis, certain treatments are recommended.

A 'cool'-energy person is offered a Melaka palm sugar and honey scrub, a hot nutmeg and rice rolling body massage, a pandan leaf and coconut milk hair mask and a unique facial that employs birds' nest saliva as its main ingredient. This is combined with a miraculously cool jade roller and a mask made from fermented tapioca. The 'warm'-energy person, on the other hand, would be encouraged to undergo a body scrub made from yoghurt and chopped guava leaves (high in natural antibiotic properties), a unique body therapy that involves rolling hard boiled eggs on the body, a calamansi lime and yoghurt hair mask, a birds' nest saliva facial and finally a mask made from fresh starfruit (*Averrhoa carambola*). Starfruit is vitamin rich and highly prized in Peranakan culture: lying with slices of cleansing, 'cooling'

starfruit doing their magic on the face is incredibly exotic.

To augment the benefits of the spa, a panel of Peranakan culinary experts has perfected a number of Nyonya specialties using this hot–cold thesis. A menu of 'cool' energy and 'warm' energy dishes using local produce and typical Peranakan herbs and spices is an innovative idea at the spa.

Such inspirational spa ideas maintain culture and tradition and give guests a highly novel experience. They are a good example of Malaysia's positioning as a spa destination with a difference.

Above Egg undulation.

Below Starfruit is vitamin rich and highly prized in Peranakan culture.

Opposite The Peranakan community adheres to a creative intermingling of Chinese and Malay traditions, resulting in a distinct culture of beauty and wellness.

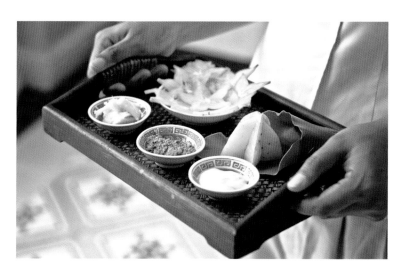

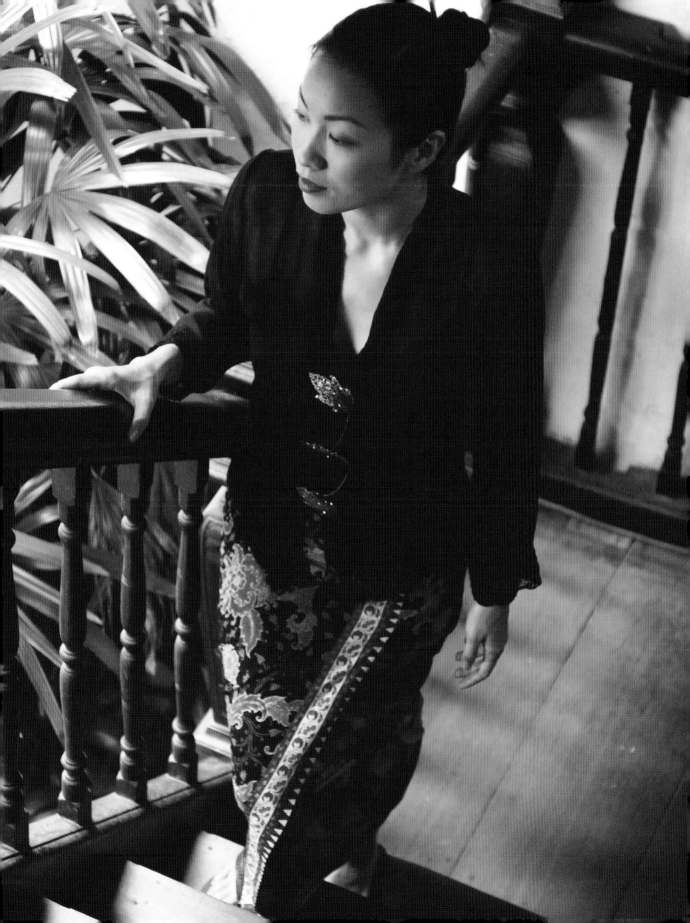

Beauty Therapies with Roots in the Imperial Courts

In the Imperial courts of the past, physicians would often come together to diagnose, devise or adapt herbal remedies and discuss their best practices. As a result there is a large collection of documented formulae for prolonging life, improving wellbeing and maintaining beauty and youthfulness; most are meant for external application, although there are a few time-tested remedies prescribed for internal consumption.

Some of these—the facials using ground pearl powder, the skin brightening lotions, the eye treatments and more—are finding their way into modern-day Malaysian spas. Some have been used at home by Malaysian Chinese for decades; others are new to the general populace, but are gaining credibility because of their long and effective history.

Wellness Remedies Derived From the Peranakan Community

The Peranakan community (also called Straits-born Chinese) is a small Southeast Asian group found predominantly in Melaka, Penang and Singapore. Creative intermingling of Chinese and Malay traditions resulted in a distinct culture of beauty and wellness. The women, or Nyonyas as they are called, were primarily home-keepers. As such, they picked up tips on simple massages and post-natal practices from the Malays, but also learnt about Chinese herbs and cuisine from their foreign elderly Chinese maids (*amah jie*).

The underlying Peranakan health principle is the classic dichotomy of 'hot' and 'cold' values associated with all things—from festivals, common foods, herbs, furniture and even crockery. In general terms, that which gives rise to increased activity, growth, brightness and warmth is 'hot' in

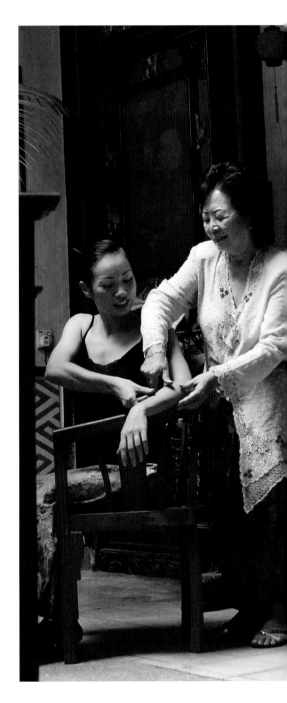

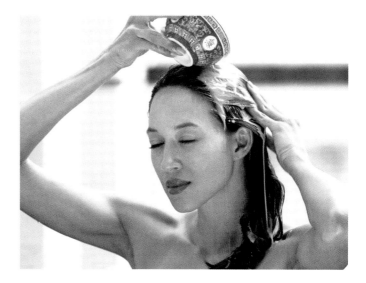

Opposite Young Nyonya girls usually learn Peranakan traditions, such as massage techniques, from the older generation.

Above Coconut milk and betel leaf hair mask.

nature, while reduced or settled activity, retardation, dimness and coolness are considered 'cold' in nature.

In the beauty and wellness sphere, different remedies were considered appropriate for 'hot' and 'cold' dispositions. For example, common rice and pearl ground into powder and mixed with a few drops of vinegar is a cooling treatment; when applied to the face, it promotes a clean, glowing complexion, especially if the face is very sensitive to heat. On the other hand, coconut milk mixed with a few betel leaves was applied on the hair after getting drenched in a heavy rainfall. A warming mask, it was applied while bathing in order to prevent a headache developing after exposure to wind, wet and cold.

Some forward-thinking spas in Malaysia have adapted some of these simple, yet profound, practices where the body is perceived in the moment as predominantly warm or cool and techniques are offered to counteract the predominance. Clients are assessed as to whether they have 'cool' or 'warm' natures, and a wellness or beauty program is suggested accordingly.

This practice allows a highly individualized interaction with clients, and, thus far, has been very well received.

A Multicultural Wellspring of Spa Possibilities

It can be seen, therefore, that traditions ranging from home care through to palace practice, from ancient systems of health and wellbeing to village folk practice—all of these play their part in the emerging Malaysian spa scenario. At its heart is the multiculturalism of Malaysian society.

While the Malay spa scene has been emerging relatively slowly on the global wellness stage, forward-looking members of the spa industry have been working with the government to actively promote the country's healing culture. Wellness tourism is a viable concern and investment in the industry is rising. As such, the Malaysian spa looks set to grow apace.

Standards for best practice are still emerging and a commitment to authenticity is needed. Master practitioners—be they highly trained exponents of their arts or village therapists whose natural gifts and family traditions have given them a deep grounding in cultural health and beauty practices—need to be identified and brought into the process. Similarly, spa operators would benefit from more ongoing training themselves.

What is clear, however, is that Malaysia, perhaps more than elsewhere in Asia, offers a collection of living traditions that is unparalleled. There is no doubt that the country has a richness of healing culture that comes from extremely diverse roots. It will undoubtedly continue to develop new and important wellness directions in the years ahead.

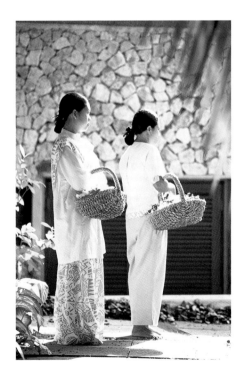

Below Attendants at a Malaysian spa resort. Cultural traditions of hospitality and warmth are enriched through ongoing professional development to ensure continual enhancement of spa standards and service.

Opposite Asia-Pacific spas numbered an estimated 21,566 in 2007.

The Global Spa Economy

In 2007, SRI International, an independent research institute in the United States, conducted an in-depth assessment of the global spa industry for the Global Spa Summit 2008 held in New York. The copyrighted data on this page is reproduced by kind permission of the Global Spa Summit 2008 (www.gss2008.org). It is especially interesting to note the high figures in the Asian sector.

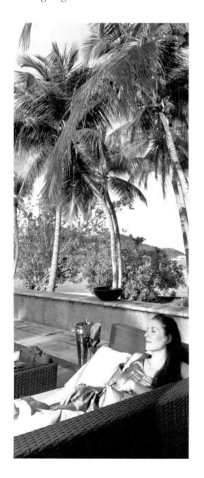

Global Spa Facilities by Region, 2007

	Estimated total number of spas	Estimated total spa revenues (US$ billion)	Estimated total spa employment
Europe	22,607	$18.4	441,727
Asia-Pacific	21,566	$11.4	363,648
North America	20,662	$13.5	307,229
Latin America–Caribbean	5,435	$ 2.5	82,694
Middle East–North Africa	1,014	$ 0.7	20,938
Africa	389	$ 0.3	7,273

Size of the Global Wellness Industry, 2007 (US$ billion)

Beauty and beauty products industry	$500.2
Fitness and fitness products industry	$241.3
Beauty and wellness medicine industry	$195.8
Healthy foods and nutrition industry	$162.4
TOTAL VALUE:	**$1,099.7**

Size of the Global Spa Industry, 2007 (US$ billion)

Core spa industry (day spas, hotel spas, destination spas, medi-spas and other spas)	$60.31
Related spa industries (spa facility operations, capital investments, spa real estate, spa education, spa consulting, spa-related hospitality and tourism)	$194.35
TOTAL VALUE:	**$254.66**

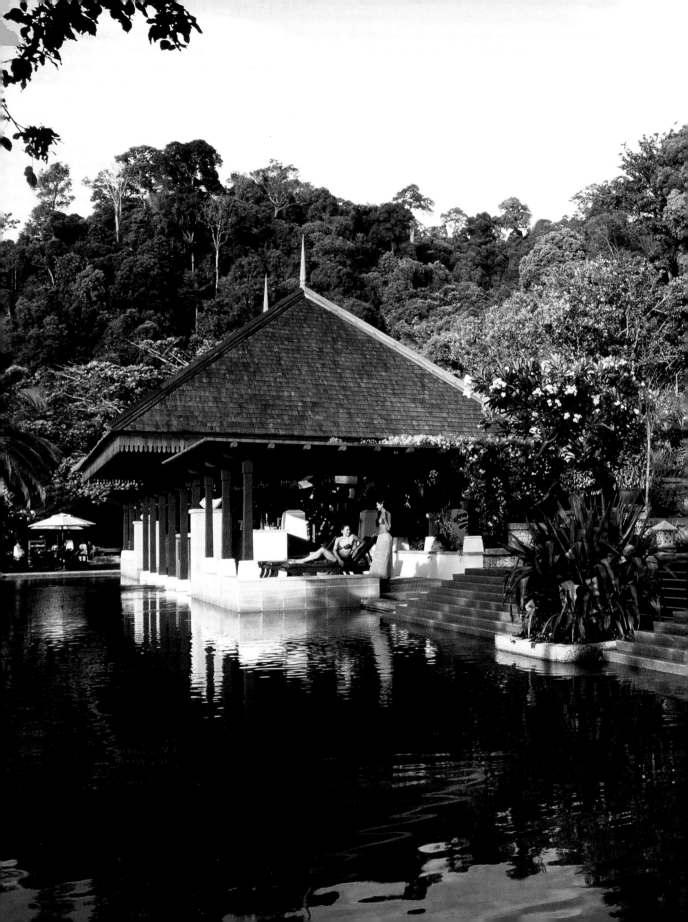

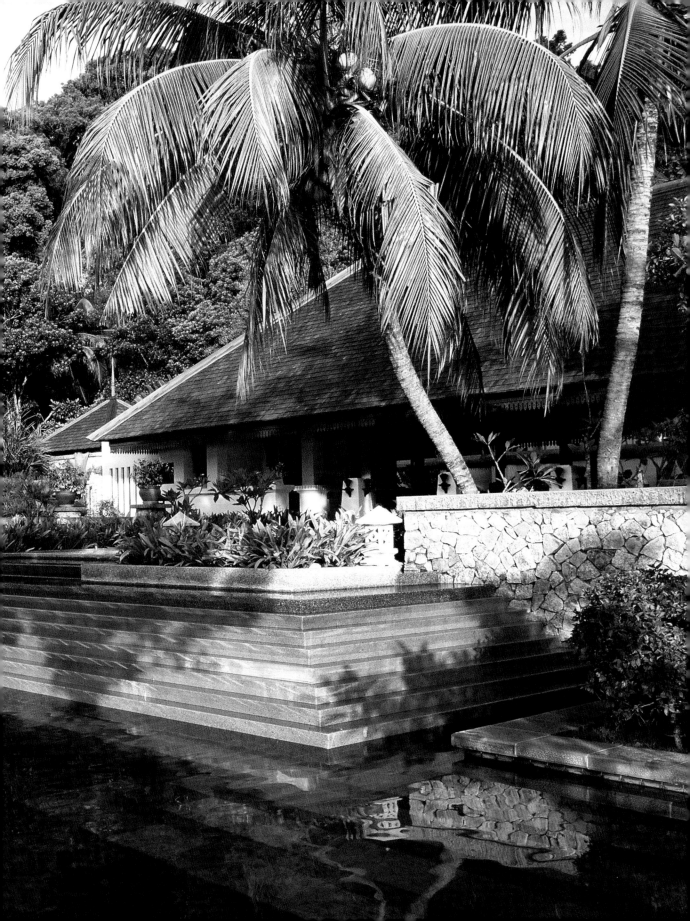

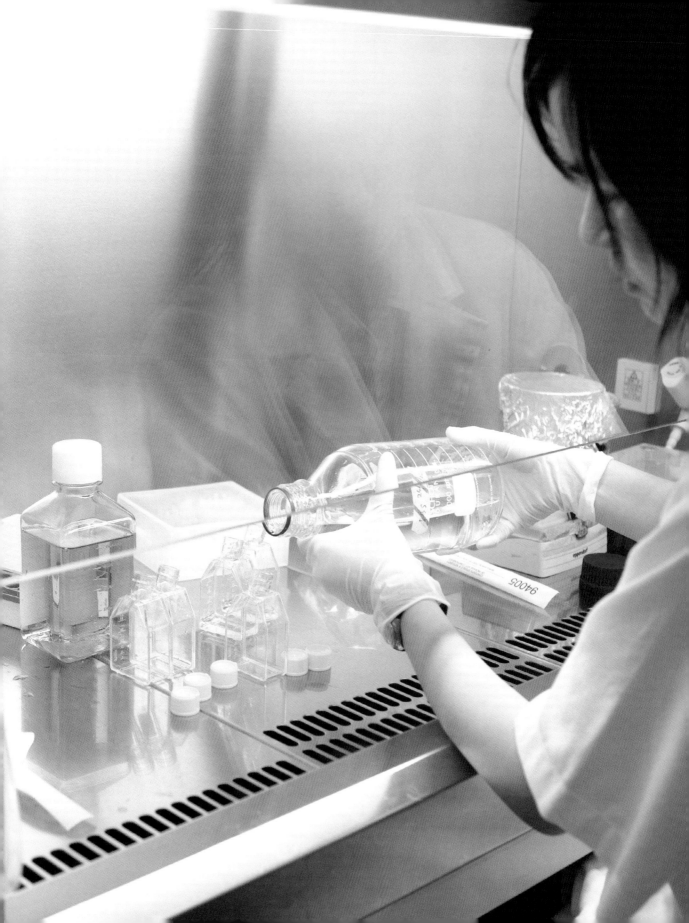

Conclusion
A Home for Malaysian Traditions in Global Wellness

The journey through time and tradition that is the *ramuan* of Malaysian health and beauty traditions reveals the substantial contribution from outsiders as well as indigenous practices. It is clear that the world has much to learn from the wisdom of the past.

Modern science is continually proving the efficacy of ancient formulations, so many in the herbal sector in Malaysia are now asking, quite reasonably: 'Where to from here?'

Today, as in the past, they want to share their herbal heritage with the world. But in what form, and how, is something that needs to be carefully considered.

> Modern science is continually proving the efficacy of ancient formulations.

Previous pages One can experience Malaysia's herbal heritage through the spa industry.

Opposite A scientist preparing cell-line cultures for bio-activity screening from Malaysia's natural resources.

The Global Herbal Market

Certainly, there is huge demand for new and important, and even exotic, healthcare products. Annual sales of herbals and supplements in the United States are currently estimated at around US$5 billion, with raw herbal materials coming increasingly from China and India. The volume of American imports of these Asian herbs now exceeds 50 percent of all global raw herbal imports. If herbal is big, Asian herbs are the biggest players within this field. Clearly, Western tastes and Eastern products are fusing in the American market.

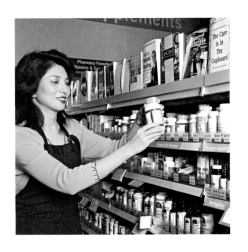

In Europe, another big importer of raw herbs from Asia, the market for herbal supplements and herbal medicines is currently worth US$7.4 billion per annum. Herbal and homeopathic medicine sales in Germany alone comprise one third of the total European market value. France, with the second highest share of the European market after Germany, is also seeing continued growth in the herbal sector.

In India, where the healthcare market is valued at around US$7.3 billion, 30 percent of drugs are now supplied by India's booming Ayurvedic industry. And in China, consumer sales in the nutrition industry are enjoying a healthy double-digit growth, reaching about US$8.1 billion in 2007. Most of this growth comes from Hong Kong and Taiwan and is linked to soaring supplement sales in vitamins and minerals, complementing a strong history in traditional Chinese medicine (TCM) products.

With Malaysia's exotic and delicious mangosteen fruit ranked at number 10 among the top-selling herbs in America, and, in 2004, with sales volume increasing by 200 percent to US$72 million, the doors to a global market are clearly opening. Noni juice, another exotic tropical fruit also found in Malaysia, saw a four percent growth increase to US$203 million in 2004.

Even so, most Malaysian herbs are still relatively unknown in international markets. Asians may know about their healing properties, with many using them regularly, but in terms of global awareness, much work needs to be done.

A number of research studies have indicated that women lead the trend in use of natural healthcare products, combining a focus on wellness, beauty, fitness and family health into new approaches to lifestyle, nutrition and herbal medicine use. Even as the global economy struggles with financial pressures, signs

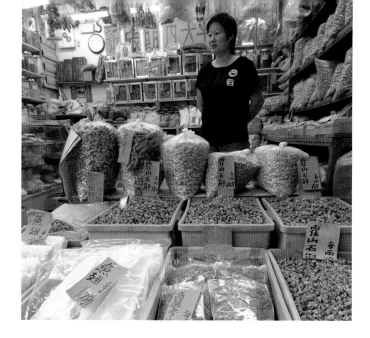

The problem lies in how to meet global demands for evidence on the safety, quality and effectiveness of herbal products.

are that healthcare in the form of self-medication and self-care remains important to women and their families. Increasingly, it is also appealing to a new and emerging group of younger men who wish to feel vital and vigorous, naturally.

These overseas markets would benefit enormously from Malaysia's chemical-free, herbal formulations. The problem lies in how to meet global demands for evidence on the safety, quality and effectiveness of herbal products. Science, naturally, plays a vital role in bringing ancient Malaysian rainforest secrets to the world stage.

Malaysia's Rich Tradition of Natural Healthcare

Looking back to the early herb and spice trade with India and China and to the precious medicinal herbs that were included more than 1,500 years ago in tributes from Malay kings to the Emperor of China, it is clear that there are centuries of continuous history of Malaysia sharing its rainforest products with the wider world. These, along with the country's health and beauty knowledge and culture, have long been 'exported' elsewhere—especially to China, India and other parts of Asia.

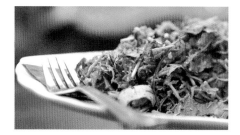

The concept of *ramuan*—the mix of healing ingredients that work together to create a new state of balance and wellbeing—is central to the local traditions of Malaysia.

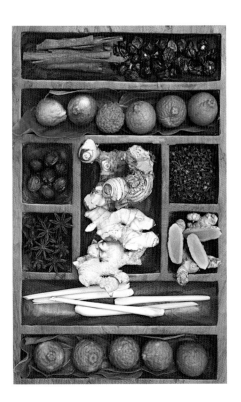

Malay medicine—with its use of *ulam* or fresh herbal salads and its combinations of herbs and spices in the form of decoctions, pastes and powders—understands well that no single component offers the key to balance. Rather, it is a wisely blended mix of discrete, powerful and compatible ingredients, all of which harness the power of healing plants from ancient tropical rainforests.

The richness of the *ramuan* tradition finds expression in nourishing, restorative and balancing Malay beauty traditions. Ingredients for complexion enhancers, herbal steam baths, massages and wraps to restore maternal health, body tone and beauty after childbirth are all drawn from field and forest; similarly, the renowned *tongkat ali* and *ubi jaga* are used to boost men's energy and vitality. All are part of a unique Asian system of healthcare found in Malaysia. Grounded in the familiar principles of humoral theory (hot and cold, damp and dry), the culture uses this framework for making sense of common ailments, for taking action to remedy these, and for restoring balance and health.

The concept of *ramuan*—the mix of healing ingredients that work together to create a new state of balance and wellbeing—is central to the local traditions of Malaysia. *Ramuan* has expanded beyond its Malay use as a mix of medicines and has come to symbolize the rich and diverse health and beauty offerings of Malaysia's many cultures.

While men focus on energy and strength, women have historically developed secret means of enhancing their beauty across the lifespan. This is one of the richest areas of the Malay medical tradition and of local forms of TCM and Ayurveda. And herein lies the promise of local traditions as they enter the world stage.

Validation of Traditional Cures through Modern Science

It is clear that in order to gain a foothold in the global herbal market, new herbal products must compete in terms of quality, safety, efficacy, pricing, and even packaging, to meet the stringent standards set by international markets.

So what are people looking for in this fiercely competitive market?

Authentic raw materials; standardized and safe extracts with zero or minimal levels of heavy metal and microbial counts; and products with reliable and stable effects.

Producers need to be able to guarantee these and, in addition, to spearhead research to satisfy both regulators and educated consumers.

Cultivation and Analysis

The research process begins with plants being brought from rainforests to ethno-botanic gardens for cultivation and further evaluation. From these collections, the best yielding plant materials can be identified and propagated for field planting.

Then, herbs are grown using the best cultivation practices and are harvested at the correct time. From these crops, when the highest quality raw materials are sent for product development, chemical analysis takes place to detect the presence of certain groups of compounds (particularly alkaloids, steroids,

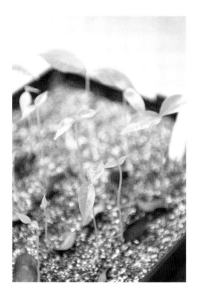

flavonoids, saponins, triterpenes and phenolic compounds).

Perfumes and Cosmetics

The extraction and analysis of essential oils is a major component in the perfume and cosmetic industry. There is a constant search for new scents and properties.

Moisture content of aromatic plant samples is first determined and then essential oils are extracted, distilled and analyzed through sophisticated processes such as (for the technically

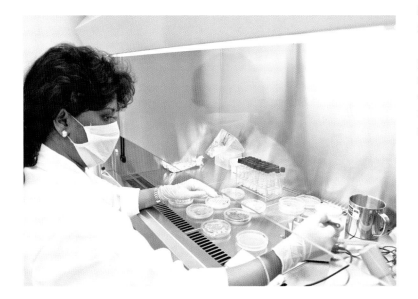

Left Selective isolation of Malaysian soil microbes—to discover, isolate and characterize potential pharmacological compounds.

Above Plants are propagated for field planting.

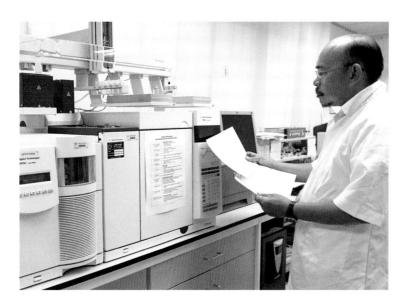

Antioxidant Properties

Of particular concern to educated consumers is whether a product can protect against the ravaging effects of oxidation on the skin, or indeed throughout the body. Oxygen, of course, is essential to all living organisms. However, oxygen is easily broken down by, for example, heat, chemical stress and ultraviolet radiation.

When oxygen does break down in this way, the resultant free radical molecules can form branching chain reactions and—like rust, which is also a free radical process—they can damage cells, DNA, proteins and fatty tissues, leading to tissue damage, injury to the immune system and symptoms of aging.

Fortunately, nature offers a solution in the form of antioxidants! Antioxidants are natural substances found in plants

Above Moisture content of plant samples are analyzed using the gas chromatography-mass spectrometry machine.

Below left Kaffir limes are cut before they are processed for their aromatic oil.

Below right Plants are tested for antioxidant properties.

Opposite Process to extract the active ingredients from plant material.

minded!) gas chromatography and gas chromatography-mass spectrometry analysis.

Once the essential oil components and molecular weights of compounds are known, the uniqueness and authenticity of the fragrance or preparation are enhanced.

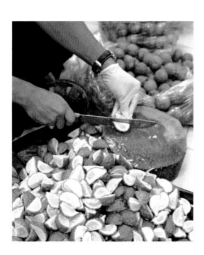

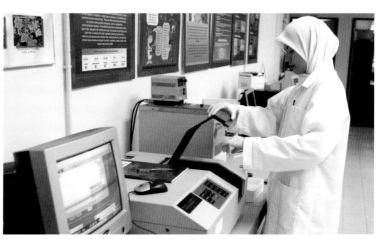

that fight and destroy excess free radicals and repair the oxidative damage that free radicals cause. New technologies can readily detect antioxidant properties in plants; and a striking number of Malaysian rainforest plants, used traditionally as medicines and medicinal foods, exhibit high concentrations of antioxidants. This is good news for the public at large as well as for producers.

Safe and High-Quality Products

Most countries have rules and regulations to ensure that herbal products are produced in safe, clean environments and that the quality of the finished herbal products is consistent and stable.

Factory processing includes washing, drying and crushing the herbs. Then, a process of extraction begins, during which the plant material is soaked in water and boiled to extract the active ingredients. After extraction, the solution is concentrated and either spray dried or freeze dried to obtain the active ingredients in a pure solid form. Then, to stabilize the product before pressing it into capsule or pill form, the active compounds are blended with fillers.

During this process a granulator (a double cone blender homogenizer) is employed

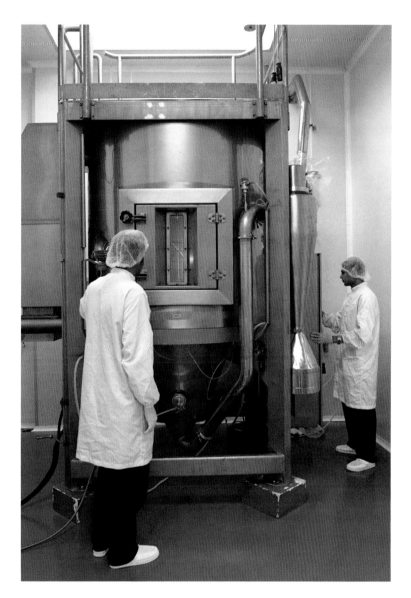

to ensure that the mixture is thoroughly mixed and uniform. The final blended mixture is then either made into capsules or pressed into tablets. At every stage of the production process,

quality control tests are carried out to ensure that the final products are clean, safe and compliant with good manufacturing practices (GMP) before the product leaves the factory.

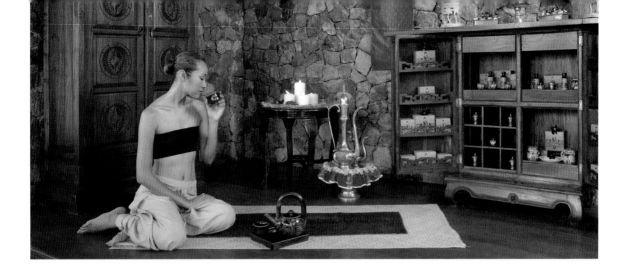

Mixing Old with New

The well informed in the herbal industry are aware that the time is right to go global. The world is increasingly using natural forms of healthcare and demand for more of the same is high. The World Health Organization's Global Atlas on Traditional Complementary and Alternative Medicine mapped these trends in 2005, showing how the rapidly growing field of natural healthcare is now becoming well established in official health policy in most countries of the world. And, of course, trade in herbal products is booming. Asian healthcare traditions are in a lead position here. Not only does Asia have the raw materials, it has the knowledge as well.

At home, Malaysia is tapping into the spa industry with the growth of Malay-, TCM- and Ayurvedic-themed spas, offering global visitors a taste of the country's ancient practices. Stress management programs are emerging as popular options for spa goers in times of global uncertainty and medical spas and healthy lifestyle programs seem more likely to flourish than those that simply focus on pampering and luxury.

At the same time that Malaysia's spas are winning global awards for their quality and uniqueness in herbal wellness, beauty treatments and exotic tropical environments, a Malaysian owned and inspired spa has opened in London's West End. It brings treatments from Malaysia and the region to discerning Londoners. And in nearby Knightsbridge, the

Above Malaysia is offering visitors a taste of the country's ancient practices through the spa industry.

Opposite Old practices—such as facial steaming—are being designed and revitalized to meet the needs of modern consumers.

luxury department store Harrods has been featuring Malay-themed spa treatments and products in recent years. Harrods fly in Malaysian spa experts and therapists to offer VIP *ramuan* treatments to the store's patrons.

Most recently, a Malaysian government-linked company has been playing a major role in the development of Malaysia's herbal industry. It has been establishing key activities—determining the active ingredients in traditional herbal preparations, conducting clinical trials on medicinally important species, creating a cutting-edge research and development platform—to build international collaborations and ensure strategic access to international markets.

Clearly, momentum is building to re-establish the prominent position that the Malay Peninsula once held as a historic center of global trade, featuring important medicinal plant exchange, between East and West.

Not only will this help to conserve species in the country's rainforests, many of which are under threat from pressures of logging, small-scale agriculture and large-scale commercial farming, it will also help to preserve the knowledge that has been guarded for so long.

As people move from the countryside to the city, adapting to life away from forest and field, the old systems are in danger of dying out. A new life of culturally familiar over-the-counter remedies and commercial beauty products may help preserve these age-old traditions by producing high-quality, safety-tested herbal products that combine the best of the old and the new. Naturally, this must be matched by recording, preserving, and revitalizing the traditions within the culture. As the West looks to the East for this knowledge, Malaysia's *ramuan* heritage is well placed to meet the demand.

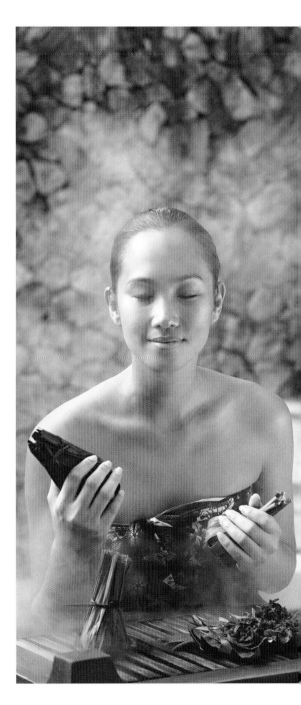

Editors' Profiles

Gerard Bodeker

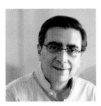

Gerard Bodeker is a senior faculty member in Public Health at Oxford University and adjunct professor of Epidemiology at Columbia University, New York. He has been chair of the Commonwealth Working Group on Traditional, Complementary and Alternative Medicine and has done work on traditional medicine and medicinal plant conservation for a number of UN agencies, including the World Health Organization, the World Bank, the Global Environment Facility and the UN Food and Agriculture Organization, for which he produced, with colleagues, a book entitled *Medicinal Plants for Forest Conservation and Healthcare*. He is founding chairman of the Oxford-based Global Initiative for Traditional Systems (GIFTS) of Health (www.giftsofhealth.org), an international research and policy partnership for the promotion and development of traditional healthcare systems. He writes and edits extensively on traditional and complementary medicine and led the editorial team that produced the *World Health Organization Global Atlas on Traditional, Complementary and Alternative Medicine*. He also co-edited a new book on understanding the global spa industry for Elsevier Press, Oxford.

Hood Salleh

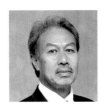

Hood Salleh is the editor of the *Peoples and Traditions* volume of *The Encyclopedia of Malaysia*. He is a professor of Medical Anthropology at Universiti Kebangsaan Malaysia (UKM) and was foundation chair of Malay Studies at Victoria University of Wellington, New Zealand from 1997 to 2000. His main fields of interest are religion and shamanism, indigenous notions of leadership and the study of climate change and the environment. He is at present an emeritus professor and principal research fellow at the Institute of Environment and Development (LESTARI) at UKM and the director of the Museum of Academic Heritage at the same university. He was rapporteur-generale for the UN World Conference on Indigenous People in 1993 and has worked for the UN Development Programme as National Steering Committee Chairman (2005–2007) on capacity building for sustainable tropical forestry among communities in Malaysia.

Ruzy Suliza Hashim

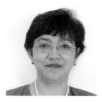

Ruzy Suliza Hashim is an associate professor at the School of Language Studies and Linguistics, Universiti Kebangsaan Malaysia. She was the chair of the School of Language Studies from 2005 to 2008. Her book, *Out of the Shadows: Women in Malay Court Narratives*, won the 2005 national book award. Her areas of interest include comparative literature and gender issues in literature. She received her Bachelor of Arts (Hons) in English from the University of Otago, New Zealand in 1986 and her PhD from the same *alma mater* in 1999. She has published extensively and supervised many postgraduate students.

Christof Jaenicke

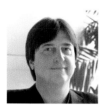

Christof Jaenicke is a physician and renowned expert on clinical nutrition. As an experienced clinician, he has held several senior management posts in leading pharmaceutical companies, with responsibility for business development and new product development, marketing and international business. He was also responsible for more than 100 clinical and pharmacological studies on phyto-pharmaceuticals, dietary supplements and medical devices in Europe, the United States, Australia and Asia. He is co-author of *Handbuch Phytotherapie*, *Physician Desk Reference for Herbal Medicine* and *Family Guide to Natural Medicines & Healing Therapies*. He is the co-founder of a world-leading consulting company focusing on natural products.

Joerg Gruenwald

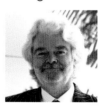

An experienced medical scientist, Joerg Gruenwald holds a doctorate in Botany and was a scientific director and head of Clinical Research of a prominent phyto-pharmaceutical company based in Berlin, Germany. He was responsible for more than 100 clinical and pharmacological studies on phyto-pharmaceuticals and dietary supplements in Europe, the United States, Australia and Asia and is the co-author of the international reference work for botanical medicines entitled *Physician Desk Reference for Herbal Medicine*. He also co-edited the *Complete German Commission E Monographs* and was editor-in-chief of *Advances in Natural Therapy*. He was a member of the United States Pharmacopeia (USP). He is an executive director of the International Kava Executive Council (IKEC) and the co-founder of a world-leading consulting company focusing on natural products.

Zurinawati Zainal Abidin

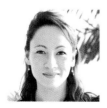

Zurinawati Zainal Abidin is the head of Corporate Communications and External Relations in a Malaysian government-linked company that researches, develops and produces natural herbal products for international markets. Her work experience has been mainly involved in coordinating and promoting the herbal industry in Malaysia. She has also been a consultant on several projects and a representative on several committees at the national level relating to the development of the country's herbal industry.

Contributors' Profiles

Daniel Baskaran

Daniel Baskaran is a former senior director of the Biotechnology Division in Forest Research Institute of Malaysia (FRIM). He received his bachelor's degree in Agriculture in 1981 from Harayana Agricultural University of India and later his master's (1983) and PhD (1986) in Seed Science from Universiti Putra Malaysia, majoring in Genetic Conservation of Tropical Recalcitrant Seeded Species. He was a member of the Malaysian Society of Plant Physiology (1990–2006) and the Malaysian Association of Research Scientists (1996–2005). His professional interest lies in medicinal and forest biotechnology.

Dorai Raja

Well known as a pioneer of Ayurveda in Malaysia since the 1980s, Dorai Raja undertook medical training at the University of Bonn in Germany, then obtained a bachelor's degree in Ayurvedic Medicine and Surgery at Patna, Bihar in India. He is the president of the Malaysian Association of Traditional Indian Medicine (MASTIM) and a key member of the Standing Committee, Traditional and Complementary Division, Ministry of Health, Malaysia. Dorai Raja is also an honorary adviser for traditional and complementary medicine policy and practice at the Ministry of Health, Malaysia, and a director at the Darshan Acupuncture and Ayurvedic Centre in Penang, Malaysia.

Andrew Forbes

With a Bachelor of Arts in Chinese Studies, a master's degree in Islamic Studies and a doctorate in Central Asian History, all from the University of Leeds, UK, Andrew Forbes is the editor and Southeast Asia correspondent of Crescent Press Agency (CPA Media Co. Ltd). Previous posts have included lecturer in History at University of Khartoum, Sudan; research fellow at the Centre of International and Area Studies, University of London; lecturer in Islamic Studies, University of Aberdeen, Scotland; and Leverhulme Fellow, British Institute in Southeast Asia, Bangkok, Thailand. He has contributed articles to many publications, including *Far Eastern Economic Review*, *The Guardian*, *The Nation*, *Wall Street Journal Europe*, *Wall Street Journal Asia*, *South China Morning Post*.

Haliza Mohd Riji

Haliza Mohd Riji teaches Medical Sociology and Anthropology in the Faculty of Medicine and Health Sciences at the Universiti Putra Malaysia (UPM). She holds a Bachelor of Arts in Sociology and Anthropology, a master's in Social Science and a doctorate in Medical Anthropology. Her recent publications include *Beauty or Health: A Personal View* (*Malaysian Family Physician*, vol. 1 (1) 2006) and *Well-being of the Elderly: Linking Objective and Subjective Dimensions in a Wellness Index* (*Brunei Journal of Health*, vol. 2, 2007). She is currently writing a book on aging and the life satisfaction of the elderly.

Hamzah Abu Al-Haj

As the CEO of the Nona Roguy Group, a company that manufactures natural herbal products, Hamzah Abu Al-Haj has been instrumental in promoting the local herbal industry and setting new scientific standards in manufacturing. He has been appointed to several national committees and is president of the Federation of Traditional Malay Medicine of Malaysia and chairman of the Malaysian Umbrella Bodies for Traditional and Complementary Medicine. In recognition of his services, he was appointed a Justice of the Peace by the Sultan of Kelantan in 1997.

Musa Yaacob

Musa Yaacob has a bachelor's degree in Agricultural Science from Massey University, New Zealand. He started working at the Malaysian Agriculture Research and Development Institute (MARDI) in 1977 as a research officer (Plant Cross Breeding). His plant focuses are roselle and herbal plants such as *tongkat ali, mas cotek*, and *dukung anak*. He is also involved in the collection of germ plasma of medicinal plants used by herbal practitioners in Malaysia. Currently, he is the assistant director for the Herbal Plants Programme at MARDI.

Sharifah Anisah Syed Agil Barakbah

Founder and chairman of the Nona Roguy Group, a company that manufactures natural herbal products, Sharifah Anisah Syed Agil Barakbah is also the author of *Ensiklopedia Perbidanan Melayu* and a book on natural childbirth practices. She is the vice-president of PUTRAMAS, an organization that represents small-scale industries in Malaysia, and a panel member of a Ministry of Health body that is compiling a standards and practices curriculum for traditional and complementary medicine production.

Lee Jok Keng

Lee Jok Keng holds a Bachelor of Arts in Psychology and a Master of Arts in Eastern Philosophy from the University of Iowa and is a member of the American Association of Oriental Medicine (AAOM), licensed to practice traditional Chinese medicine (TCM) in the United States. He is also registered with Malaysia's Ministry of Health as a TCM practitioner. He has been actively involved in TCM for the last 30 years, and presently heads his own consulting company, Gaia Matrix Solutions, a TCM resource provider. He designed and provided therapist training for some of the spas owned and operated by the YTL Group and develops herbal formulations for Eu Yan Sang. Jok Keng is also a member of the advisory board for SpaAsia Wellness Media Ltd.

Sairani Mohd Sa'ad

A certified trainer and consultant for traditional Malay treatments at the Persatuan Perubatan Tradisional Melayu Malaysia and Nona Roguy, Sairani Mohd Sa'ad is also a Consultant and Trainer for the YTL Group, with the responsibility for establishing a menu of traditional Malay treatments in the spas at Pangkor Laut Resort, Tanjong Jara Resort, the Ritz-Carlton and Cameron Highlands Resort. She has travelled extensively to promote Malay therapies at Urban Retreats, Harrods, London as well as venues in Paris, Hawaii, Las Vegas and other Asian countries. She is working on the structure of a bachelor's course in Malay Medicine in the Traditional and Complementary Medicine Division of the Ministry of Health.

Zainatul Shuhaida Abdul Rahman

Head editor of Zebra Editions Sdn Bhd, Zainatul Shuhaida Abdul Rahman was instrumental in the setting up of the magazine *Herba & Perubatan* (Herbs & Medicine). The aim of the magazine is to educate and inform readers about Malaysia's rich traditions of herbal healing. The magazine, now in its 11th volume, contains articles—featuring pictures and interviews—compiled first hand by Shuhaida.

Glossary

Abhyanga (uh-be-ung-ga) Ayurvedic massage applied according to a daily or seasonal regime

Adat (uh-dut) Traditional social custom, law

Akar (uh-kar) Root

Ama (um-maa) Body waste or toxins

Amah jie (um-uh jee) Chinese maid or helper

An-mo (un-moh) Chinese 'press and rub' massage

Anak rambut (uh-nuck rum-boot) Fine hair that grows on the fringe of the forehead

Andaman (un-duh-mun) Bridal grooming

Angin (uh-ngeen) Wind, air

Asana (uh-suh-nuh) Yoga posture, the third stage in Yoga

Ayurveda (eye-yoor-vey-duh) Classical Vedic science of health and wellbeing

Baba (buh-buh) Male Straits-born Chinese (Peranakan)

Balgam / balgham (bul-gum) Mucus, phlegm

Banyak angin (buh-nyuk uh-ngeen) Excess of wind

Barut (buh-root) Body-binding, body-wrapping

Batin (buh-teen) Concealed, inner, hidden

Bedak sejuk (beh-duck seh-jook) Cooling 'pearl' powder made from rice

Belachan / belacan (beh-luh-chun) Fermented shrimp paste

Benang mentah (beh-nung mehn-tuh) Unprocessed thread

Bengkung (behng-kong) Body-binding

Berdiang (behr-dee-yung) Sauna; to heat on a warm fire

Berinai (behr-ee-nigh) To apply henna

Berpantang (behr-pun-tung) Malay post-natal care

Bersanding (behr-sun-deeng) Malay wedding custom during which the couple sit together on a dais

Bertangas kering (behr-tung-us ker-eeng) Herbal dry sauna

Bertih (behr-teeh) Rice fried in the husk

Bertimpuh (behr-teem-poh) Polite sitting posture in the Malay tradition

Bertuam (behr-too-wum) Hot compress to reduce pain made using heated objects wrapped with cloth

Bertungku (behr-toong-koo) Hot iron compress

Bhuta (boo-tuh) Element

Bidan (bee-dun) Malay midwife, therapeutic masseur

Bomoh (boh-moh) Malay traditional medicine man, healer

Bomoh patah (boh-moh puh-tuh) Traditional Malay healer specializing in bone setting

Buang cangrai (boo-wung chung-rye) Casting away ill luck

Buka urat (boo-ka oo-rut) Massage technique that 'strokes towards the heart'

Bunga (boo-nguh) Flower

Burut (boo-root) Hernia

Burut tarik (boo-root tuh-reek) A form of viscous wind

Buyung (boo-yoong) Earthenware pot

Candi (chan-dee) Ancient Hindu-Buddhist temple

Cepu (cheh-poo) Small ornamental casket

Champi (chum-pee) Ayurvedic head massage

Charaka Samhita (chu-rah-kah sung-hee-tuh) Preeminent Ayurvedic text

Cukur jambul (choo-koor jum-bowl) Malay head-shaving ceremony for newborn babies

Cupak (choo-puck) A cubic measure

Darah (duh-ruh) Blood

Daun (duh-woon) Leaf

Demam (deh-mum) Fever, ague

Dhara (duh-rah) Pouring of herbal liquids on body parts

Dhatu (duh-too) Body tissue

Dhyan (dee-yun) Yogic meditation

Dieda (tee-yeyh-duh) Traditional Chinese 'hit and fall medicine'

Dinacharya (dee-nuh-chuh-ree-ya) Ayurvedic daily regime

Doa (doe-uh) Islamic prayer invoking a blessing

Dosha (doe-shuh) Ayurvedic principle of physiology

Dukun (doo-koon) Malay healer, herbalist, soothsayer

Gamat (guh-mut) Sea cucumber

Garam janta (guh-rum jun-tun) A kind of coarse salt

Hari (huh-ree) Day

Harian (huh-ree-yun) Daily

Hatha yoga (hath-uh-yoh-guh) Type of yoga that focuses on physical movement

Ibu (ee-boo) Mother, source

Ibu ubat (ee-boo oo-but) Mother of medicine

Ikan (ee-kun) Fish

Ikan haruan (ee-kun huh-roo-wun) Striped snakehead fish

Jiecha (jee-yey chuh) Old Chinese name for Kedah

Kadaram (Kuh-duh-rum) Ancient Indian name for Kedah

Kain (Kuh-yen / kuh-yeen) Cloth, sarong

Kalah (kuh-luh) Old Arabic name for Kedah

Kampung (kum-pong) Malay village

Kapha (kuh-ffuh) Water element in Ayurveda; the principle of structure or preservation

Karma (kuhr-muh) Action

Kayu (kuh-you) Wood

Kembung perut (kehm-boong per-root) Flatulence

Kunci (koon-chee) Silat term used to describe a 'lock'

Langit-langit mulut (luh-ngeet luh-ngeet moo-loot) The palate or roof of the mouth

Lemah semangat (leh-muh seh-muh-ngut) Weak life force, spirit; to feel faint

Lendiran angin (len-dyr-run uh-ngeen) Viscous wind

Lenguh (leh-ngooh) Aches and pains

Lintah (leen-tuh) Leech

Luar gelanggang (loo-wur geh-lung-gung) Silat term meaning 'outside the arena'

Lulut (loo-loot)   Body scrub

Lulut wangi (loo-loot wung-ee)   Scented body scrub

Maha (muh-huh)   Great, mighty

Majun (muk-joon)   Herbal tonic

Majun kuat (muk-joon koo-wut)   Bitter herbal tonic

Mak andam (muk un-dum)   Malay bridal attendant

Mandi (mun-dee)   Bath, bathing

Mandi bunga puteri (mun-dee boong-uh poo-teh-ree)
    Princess's floral bath

Mandi embun (mun-dee em-bone)   Dew bath

Mandi limau (mun-dee lee-mao)   Kaffir lime bath

Mandi rempah (mun-dee rhem-puh)   Herbal spice bath

Mandi wap (mun-dee wup)   Steam bath, sauna

Mandul (mun-dool)   Infertility

Mantah wangi (mun-tuh wung-ee)   Floral elixir

Mantera (mun-truh)   Mantra, invocation

Marma (muhr-muh)   Ayurvedic system of energy points
    for healing body, mind and consciousness

Mati pucuk (muh-tee poo-chook)   Impotence

Meroyan (meh-ro-yun)   Postpartum depression, mother's blues

Minyak (mee-nyuk)   Oil

Minyak attar (mee-nyuck uh-tar)   Non-alcoholic perfume made
    from agarwood that is applied to Muslim prayer clothes

Muppini (moo-pee-nee)   Theory of five elements and
    three *doshas*

Nikah (nee-kuh)   Malay wedding solemnization

Nyonya (nyo-nyuh)   Female Straits-born Chinese (Peranakan)

Ojas (oh-jus)   Indian term for vigor and vitality; a subtle and
    vital fluid that is the essence of all tissue

Orang Asli (oh-rung us-lee)   Indigenous peoples of Malaysia

Panas (puh-nuss)   Heat, hot

Panchakarma (puhn-chuh kahr-muh)   A five-fold eliminative
    therapy in Ayurveda, facilitating a complete cleansing
    through the natural eliminatory pathways of the body

Panchamahabhuta (pan-chuh-muh-hub-boo-tuh)   Five great
    organizing principles described in Vedic science

Pantang larang (pun-tung luh-rung)   Prohibitions and taboos

Paschatkarma (pass-chut-kahr-muh)   Post-treatment care
    in Ayurveda

Pawang (puh-wung)   Shaman, magician, mystical specialist

Pengapit (peh-nguh-peet)   Matron of honor

Penyakit (peh-nyuh-keet)   Illness or disease

Penyakit angin pasang (peh-nyuh-keet uh-ngeen puh-sung)   Bad
    wind ailments

Penyakit melanuih (peh-nyuh-keet muh-laa-noo-weeh)
    Premenopausal syndrome

Peranakan (pehr-ruh-nuh-kun)   Straits-born Chinese

Periuk (pehr-ree-yook)   A cooking pot

Petua (peh-too-wuh)   Folk wisdom

Pitam (pee-tum)   A rush of blood to the head causing dizziness

Pitta (pit-tuh)   Ayurvedic fire or metabolic principle; one
    of the three *doshas* governing bodily functions

Pokok (poh-kock)   Tree

Pradhanakarma (pruh-dah-nuh-kahr-muh)   Ayurvedic
    main treatment

Pranayama (pruh-nuh-yuh-muh)   Science of breath control

Pucuk (poo-chook)   Young shoots of plants or herbs

Pukul (poo-kool) Term used in silat to describe a 'strike'

Pulih semangat (poo-leeh seh-muh-ngut) Returning life spirit

Purvakarma (poor-vah-kahr-muh) Different types of continuous oil massages and fomentation

Qi (chee) Chinese concept of life force

Qigong (chee gong) Ancient Chinese healthcare system that integrates physical postures, breathing techniques and focused intentions

Ramu / ramuan (ruh-moo, ruh-moo-wun) Ingredients, things; therapeutic formulations from mixtures of medicinal herbs and plants

Ramu tenaga batin (ruh-moo teh-nuh-guh buh-teen) Herbal mixture for vitality and libido

Ramuan akar kayu (ruh-moo-wun ah-car kuh-yoo) Herbal root mixture

Ramuan asli (ruh-moo-wun us-lee) Original herbal mixture

Rawatan (ruh-wuh-tun) Treatment, therapy

Rawatan gamat (ruh-wuh-tun guh-mut) Sea cucumber treatment

Rempah (rhem-puh) Spices, ingredients

Rempah ratus (rhem-puh ruh-toos) Poly-herbal preparations

Rendam herba (rhen-dum her-buh) Herbal immersion, herbal sitz bath

Resdong (resh-dong) Sinusitis

Ritucharya (ree-too-chuh-ree-ya) Ayurvedic seasonal routine

Sakit (suh-keet) Sick, diseased, unwell

Sakit-sakit (suh-keet suh-keet) Aches and pains

Sanskrit (san-skreet) Classical language of Northern India

Santan (sun-tun) Coconut milk

Sejuk (seh-jook) Cold, damp

Senaman asak badan (seh-nuh-mun uh suk buh-dun) Therapeutic Malay exercises

Seri (seh-ree) Aura, charm

Senaman harimau (seh-nuh-mun huh-ree-mao) 'Tiger posture' exercise

Senaman ular (seh-nuh-mun oo-lur) 'Snake posture' exercise

Seribu bunga (seh-ree-boo boong-uh) Thousand flower essence

Shirodhara (she-rod-hara) Ayurvedic treatment with herbal oil poured on forehead

Shiva (she-vuh) Hindu deity of purification and dissolution

Siddha (see-duh) Classical Tamil healthcare system of South India

Siddhar (see-duhr) Masters of the Siddha healthcare tradition

Siddhi (seed-dhee) Perfection

Silat (see-lut) Malay martial art

Sinseh (seen-sayh) Traditional Chinese herbalist, medicine man

Sirih (see-rayh) betel leaf

Suci murni (soo-chee moor-nee) Malay concept of purity of spirit, health and general wellbeing

Suvarnabhumi (soo-vuhr-nuh-boo-mee) Sanskrit term for 'golden land', applied to the ancient region including Kadaram

Sweda (sway-duh) Sweat

Swedanam (sway-duh-num) Ayurvedic sweat therapy

Tai chi (Tai-ji / tie-chee) Chinese system of physical exercise for meditation and self-defense

Tamilakam (Thamil-uk-um) An ancient Indian dynasty

Tangas kering (tung-ngus keh-reeng) Dry herbal sauna

TCM Traditional Chinese medicine

Tepak sirih (tay-puk see-rayh) Betel quid container

Teruk (teh-rook) Severe, serious, chronic

Tok batin (toock buh-teen) Proto-Malay tribal chief

Tok guru silat (toock goo-roo see-lut) Silat master

Tri dosha (tree-doe-shuh) Ayurvedic three dosas

Tuam pasir (too-wum puh-syr) Application of dry heat in the form of a bag of hot sand or bran

Tuaman (too-wum-mun) Compress

Tuaman batu (too-wum-mun buh-too) Hot stone compress

Tui-na (too-wee nuh) Chinese 'push and hold' massage

Tungku batu (toong-koo buh-too) Stone in the hearth

Tutup urat (too-toop oo-rut) Massage technique with 'strokes away from the heart'

Ubat (oo-but) Medicine, pharmaceutical

Ubat barut (oo-but buh-root) Medicated body-binding ointment

Ubat mantah (oo-but mun-tuh) Fresh herbal decoction

Ubat mantah wangi (oo-but mun-tuh wung-ngee) Fresh aromatic herbal decoction

Ubat periuk (oo-but pehr-ree-yook) Herbal tonic drink for internal cleansing and health

Ujud anggota (oo-jood uhng-go-tuh) Life force of the human body; soul

Ukup (oo-koop) Sauna, body steaming

Ukup kering (oo-koop kehr-reeng) Dry herbal steam

Ukup rempah (oo-koop rehm-puh) Spicy body steam

Ukup wangi (oo-koop wung-ngee) Sweet-scented sauna

Ulam (oo-lum) Raw herbal salad

Upacara naik seri (oo-puh-char-uh nuh-yeek seh-ree) Aura-enhancement ceremony

Upacara semangat sirih (oo-puh-char-uh seh-muh-ngut see-rayh) Spirit of the betel leaf ceremony

Upacara tijak bumi (oo oo-puh-char-uh tee-juk boo-mee) Baby 'earth-stepping' ceremony

Urat (oo-rut) Veins, arteries

Urut (oo-root) Massage, rub with the hands

Urut Melayu (oo-root meh-luh-yoo) Malay massage

Urutan asak (oo-roo-tun uh-suk) Therapeutic massage

Urutan bayi (oo-roo-tun buh-yee) Baby massage

Urutan sengkak (oo-roo-tun sehng-kuk) Full-body massage to reposition the uterus

Urutan sentuhan (oo-roo-tun sehn-too-hun) Type of massage for the stomach and to loosen tense muscles

Urutan tenaga batin (oo-roo-tun teh-nuh-guh buh-teen) Traditional massage for vitality, manhood massage

Urutan tuaman batu (oo-roo-tun too-wum-mun buh-too) Hot stone massage

Vaidya (vite-hya) Ayurvedic physician

Vata (vuh-tuh) Wind element in Ayurveda

Vatsu (vus-too) Vedic system of architecture

Vedic (vay-deek) Early Sanskrit in which the Vedas are written

Xian sheng (See-yen sheng) Mandarin term used to address a medicine man, herbalist or any learned or elderly person

Yin-yang (ying-yung) Traditional Chinese philosophy to describe inner energy and physical balance

Yoga (yoh-guh) Classical Indian system of mind–body integration

Yogas chitta vritti nirodhaha (yoh-gus chit-tah vr-tee nee-ro-da-ha) A 'settled state of mind' in Ayurvedic tradition

Zahir (zuh-heer) Clear, manifest, open

Zahir batin (zuh-heer buh-teen) Psycho-physical acts

Botanical Glossary

Local name	Scientific name	Other names
Akar gegerit besi	*Willughbeia edulis*	—
Akar lalang	*Imperata cylindrica*	Lalang roots
Akar semalu	*Mimosa pudica*	Touch-me-not roots
Akar serapat	*Parameria polyneura*	—
Akar wangi	*Chrysopogon zizanioides*	Vetiver roots
Amalaka / amala	*Emblica officinalis*	*Amla / amlaka / amlika* / Indian gooseberry
Asam jawa	*Tamarindus indica*	Tamarind
Asam keping / gelugor	*Garcinia atroviridis*	Garcinia
Asam susur	*Hibiscus sabdariffa*	Roselle
Belimbing	*Averrhoa carambola*	Carambola / starfruit
Bintangor	*Calophyllum* spp.	—
Bringhraj	*Eclipta alba*	Urang aring / dyer's weed
Buah keras	*Aleurites moluccana*	Candlenut
Buah pala	*Myristica fragrans*	Nutmeg
Bunga kantan	*Etlingera elatior*	Torch ginger
Bunga melur	*Jasminum sambac*	Jasmine
Bunga pakma / padma	*Rafflesia* spp.	Rafflesia
Bunga raya	*Hibiscus rosa-sinensis*	Hibiscus
Bunga susung	*Ervatamia divaricata*	—

Local name	Scientific name	Other names
Bunga tahi ayam	*Lantana camara*	Lantana
Bunga tanjung / mengkula	*Mimusops elengi* L.	Bullet-wood tree
Cabai jawa	*Piper retrofractum*	Java long pepper
Cekur	*Kaempferia galanga* Linn.	*Kencur*
Cekur manis	*Sauropus albicans*	Star gooseberry
Cempaka	*Michelia champaca*	Champak
Cengkih	*Syzygium aromaticum*	Clove
Cili padi	*Capsicum frutescens*	Bird's eye chilies
Dang shen	*Codonopsis pilosula*	Codonopsis root / false ginseng
Daun bangun-bangun	*Plectranthus amboinicus*	Indian borage
Daun baru Cina	*Artemesia vulgaris*	Moxa leaves
Daun Cina maki	*Cassia angustifolia*	Senna / senna maki / Tinnevelly senna
Daun gajus / janggus	*Anacardium occidentale*	Cashew nut leaves
Daun kari	*Murraya koenigii*	Curry leaf
Daun kesum	*Persicaria tenella*	Vietnamese coriander / *laksa* leaves
Daun ketih/turi	*Sesbania grandiflora*	—
Daun mambu	*Azadirachta indica*	Neem leaves
Daun pandan	*Pandanus odorus*	Pandanus / pandan leaves
Daun tenggek burung	*Euodia ridleyi*	*Evodia*
Dukung anak	*Phyllanthus niruri*	Stonebreaker
Gaharu / karas / jinkoh	*Aquilaria malaccensis*	Agarwood / aloeswood
Gambir	*Uncaria gambir*	Gambier
Gelang pasir	*Portulaca oleracea*	Common purslane
Halba	*Trigonella foenum graecum*	Fenugreek
Halia	*Zingiber officinale*	Ginger

Local name	Scientific name	Other names
Halia bara	*Zingiber officinale* var. rubrum	Red ginger
Hempedu bumi	*Andrographis paniculata*	Creat
Jambu	*Psidium guajava*	Guava
Janda merana	*Salix babylonica*	Willow leaves
Jarak	*Ricinus communis*	Castor oil plant
Jemuju	*Carum copticum*	Ajwain
Jerang	*Dracaena cinnabari*	Dragon's blood
Jerangau	*Acorus calamus*	Sweet flag
Jintan hitam	*Nigella sativa*	Black seed
Kaca piring	*Gardenia augusta*	Gardenia
Kacang kelang	*Clitoria ternatea* L.	Butterfly pea flower
Kacip fatimah	*Labisia pumila*	—
Kaduk	*Piper sarmentosum*	Wild betel leaf
Kayu manis	*Cinnamomum verum*	Cinnamon
Kecubung	*Datura alba*	Thorn apple
Kelapa	*Cocos nucifera*	Coconut
Kemboja	*Plumeria acuminate*	Frangipani
Kemenyan Arab	*Boswellia sacra*	Frankincense
Kemenyan Jawa	*Styrax benzoin / S. paralleloneurum*	Styrax / benzoin
Kemunting Cina	*Catharanthus roseus*	Rosy periwinkle
Kenanga	*Cananga odorata*	Ylang-ylang
Karanda	*Carissa carandas*	Golden gardenia
Keremak	*Alternanthera sessilis* L.	Carpet weed
Kesidang	*Vallaris pergulana* Burm.	—
Ketapang	*Terminalia catappa*	Sea almond

Local name	Scientific name	Other names
Ketumbit	*Leucas aspera*	—
Kuinin / kuina	*Cinchona officinalis*	Cinchona / quinine
Kulat kayu	*Ganoderma lucidum*	*Lingzhi*
Kunyit	*Curcuma longa*	Turmeric
Lada hitam	*Piper nigrum* L.	Black pepper
Lempoyang wangi	*Zingiber aromaticum*	Zerumbet ginger
Lemuni	*Vitex negundo*	Negundo chastetree
Lengkuas	*Languas galanga*	Galangal
Limau bali / limau besar	*Citrus grandis*	Pomelo
Limau batu	*Aegle marmelos*	Stone apple
Limau purut	*Citrus hystrix*	Kaffir lime
Manggis	*Garcinia mangostana*	Mangosteen
Manjakani	*Cympsgallae tinctoria*	Oak galls
Mas cotek	*Ficus deltoidea*	Mistletoe fig
Mengkudu	*Morinda citrifolia*	Noni / Indian mulberry
Mengkunyit	*Coscinium blumeanum*	False calumba
Merunggai	*Moringa oleifera*	Drumstick tree
Misai kucing	*Orthosiphon stamineus*	Java tea
Nilam	*Pogostemon cablin*	Patchouli
Patawali / pakhawali	*Tinospora cordifolia*	Guduchi / heartleaf moonseed
Patah tulang	*Cissus quadrangularis*	—
Pegaga	*Centella asiatica*	Gotu kola / Asiatic pennywort
Petai	*Parkia speciosa* Hassk.	Malayan stink bean
Pinang	*Areca catechu*	Areca nut / betel nut
Pisang kelat	*Musa acuminata*	Wild banana

Local name	Scientific name	Other names
Pokok kapal terbang	*Chromolaena odorata*	Siam weed
Pokok ketumpangan air	*Peperomia pellucida*	Shining bush
Pokok tunjuk langit	*Helminthostachys zeylanica*	Centipede plant
Sagu	*Metroxylon sagus*	Sago
Sambung nyawa	*Gynura procumbens*	—
Selasih	*Ocimum basilicum*	Sweet basil
Selasih hitam	*Ocimum tenuiflorum* L.	Holy basil / *tulsi*
Senduduk	*Melastoma malabathricum*	Singapore rhododendron
Senduduk putih	*Melastoma imbricatum*	White rhododendron
Sepang	*Caesalpinia sappan*	Sappan tree
Serai	*Cymbopogon citratus*	Lemongrass
Serai wangi	*Cymbopogon nardus*	Citronella
Setawar halia	*Costus speciosus*	Crepe ginger
Sintok	*Cinnamomum sintoc*	Sintoc
Sirih	*Piper betle*	Betel
Sundal malam	*Polianthes tuberosa*	Tuberose
Temu ireng	*Curcuma aeruginosa*	—
Temu kunci	*Gastrochilus panduratum*	*Kachai* (Thai)
Temu lawak	*Curcuma xanthorrhiza* Roxb.	Java turmeric
Temu pauh	*Curcuma mangga*	Mango ginger
Terung meranti / terung perat	*Solanum nigrum*	Black nightshade
Timba tasik	*Adenosma capitatum*	—
Tongkat ali	*Eurycoma longifolia*	Longjack
Ubi jaga	*Smilax myosotiflora*	Smilax
Ulam raja	*Cosmos caudatus*	Wild cosmos / 'king's salad'

Index

Picture Credits

All of the images in this book were photographed by S.C. Shekar, with the exception of the following:

Arkib Negara Malaysia 16, 31 (top), reprinted from *History of the Dutch in Malaysia* by Dennis De Witt, published by Nutmeg Publishing.

Asian Civilisations Museum, Singapore 36.

Gerard Bodeker 136, 137.

Bridgeman Art Library 135 (top).

British Library 156.

Corbis 150, 151, 174–175, 218 (bottom).

Martin Cross 12.

Edm Archives 15, 17, 18 (top, bottom), 19, 30 (bottom), 40 (bottom), 120, 121, 122, 123 (top left, bottom left), 133 (bottom), 154 (bottom), 155, 168, 169 (bottom).

Federal Land Development Authorities (FELDA) 30 (top), 39, 69 (bottom), 94 (bottom left, middle), 95 (bottom), 100 (top), 102 (bottom), 112 (top), 129 (top right), 158 (top, bottom left), 162 (bottom left), 194 (bottom left).

Susan Flint 134.

Mary Evans Picture Library 157 (top).

Mustaffa Mahmood
31 (bottom), 35, 41 (bottom right), 68, 69 (top), 81, 85, 88 (top), 94 (bottom right), 95 (top), 98 (bottom left), 99, 100 (bottom left, bottom right), 101 (middle), 102, 108 (top right), 110 (top), 124 (bottom), 128 (top), 129 (bottom), 139 (bottom left, top), 144 (top).

National Library Board, Singapore and Chung Chee Kit 152.

New Straits Times Press (Malaysia) Bhd 28 (top, bottom), 37.

NHPA Limited, UK 114-115, 118.

Photo Library 41 (top, bottom left), 77 (top), 111 (top), 113 (top), 123 (right), 126, 133 (top), 139 (bottom right), 157 (bottom), 158 (bottom right), 166 (bottom), 173, 200, 226-227, 230, 231 (top).

Picture Library Sdn Bhd 10-11, 12, 14, 30 (second from top), 31 (second from top), 34, 38, 77 (bottom), 89 (top), 90, 92, 93, 98 (top), 101 (top, bottom), 111 (bottom), 113 (bottom left, right), 116, 125, 138 (bottom), 142, 143, 144 (bottom), 159, 160 (right), 162 (bottom right), 163 (top), 164, 169 (top).

Sharifah Anisah Syed Agil Barakbah 43.

Star Publications (Malaysia) Bhd 21, 119, 173.

Tai Lung Aik 124 (top).

The Wellcome Library, London 135 (bottom), 153, 154 (top), 163 (bottom), 205 (top), 218 (top).

YTL Hotels and Properties Sdn Bhd 22, 23, 176, 179, 184, 185, 188, 190, 191, 193, 206 (top), 208, 212, 216 (bottom), 217 (top), 219, 220 (bottom), 223, 224, 225, 232, 236, 237.

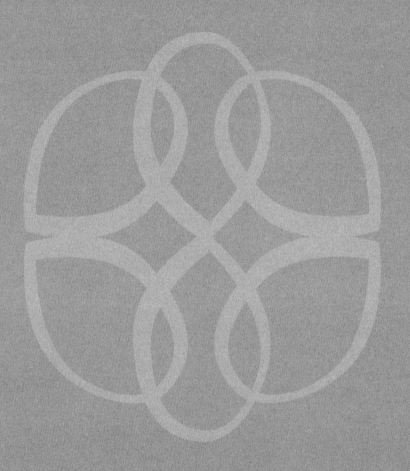